RIGHTS, RISKS AND RESPONSIBILITIES

Other books edited by Georgina Koubel and Hilary Bungay

The Challenge of Person-Centred Care: An Interprofessional Perspective (2009)

Rights, Risks and Responsibilities

Interprofessional Working in Health and Social Care

Edited by

Georgina Koubel
and
Hilary Bungay

palgrave
macmillan

First published 2012 by
PALGRAVE MACMILLAN

Palgrave Macmillan in the UK is an imprint of Macmillan Publishers Limited,
registered in England, company number 785998, of Houndmills, Basingstoke,
Hampshire RG21 6XS.

Palgrave Macmillan in the US is a division of St Martin's Press LLC,
175 Fifth Avenue, New York, NY 10010.

Palgrave Macmillan is the global academic imprint of the above companies
and has companies and representatives throughout the world.

Palgrave® and Macmillan® are registered trademarks in the United States,
the United Kingdom, Europe and other countries

ISBN-13: 978–0–230–28288–9

This book is printed on paper suitable for recycling and made from fully
managed and sustained forest sources. Logging, pulping and manufacturing
processes are expected to conform to the environmental regulations of the
country of origin.

A catalogue record for this book is available from the British Library.

A catalog record for this book is available from the Library of Congress.

10   9   8   7   6   5   4   3   2   1
21 20 19 18 17 16 15 14 13 12

Printed in China

Contents

Notes on Contributors

The majority of the contributors are fully involved in teaching, research and/or development of programmes in interprofessional education and all have experience of working interprofessionally.

The backgrounds of the contributors include a number of people with extensive experience and diverse qualifications in social work and health care, and with a variety of areas of expertise.

Adrian Adams, PhD, MSc, BA, CQSW, Head of Department Social Work, Community and Mental Health. I worked as a social worker, training coordinator and CCETSW education adviser prior to entering the university initially as a lecturer in the social work team. I have researched and published on international, interprofessional and interorganisational aspects of health and social services. There have been publications on a wide range of relevant topics including, among others, European social work and the benefits of partnership working in Europe, the modernisation of social work practice, the history of social work in the UK and the relationship between theory and practice in interprofessional education.

Jane Arnott, MSc in Health Education and Health Promotion. I have a nursing background, with three professional qualifications – a registered nurse, midwife and health visitor. I have also worked as a lecturer in a Further Education College for five years and as an education manager in a primary care trust. I worked as a health visitor for 20 years in different areas of Kent. I currently work as a senior lecturer in community nursing and continue to work with colleagues across departments in order to learn from others about professional perspectives, values and beliefs to inform my professional understanding.

I have written texts about the rights of individuals and professionals and the tensions in balancing these in the UK's contemporary health and social care arena. I am currently researching the meaning of the place in the delivery of person-centred care and have been contracted to write a book about nursing in the community.

Cathy Bernal, Senior Lecturer in Learning Disability. My background prior to taking my current post was in working with people with severe and often complex learning disabilities, and I have witnessed many times the effects of the social exclusion which is often the fate of such individuals. Since entering academia, I have taught widely on the topic of learning disability and collaboration within interprofessional education in health and social care, and worked with local learning disability services, particularly those supporting profoundly disabled people, in order to improve their person-centred responses. I have published chapters and articles on a range of subjects concerning learning disability.

Hilary Bungay PhD, Senior Lecturer in Interprofessional Learning at Anglia Ruskin University. My research interests are diverse and include the health of older people, the potential role of the arts in health and well-being, and the organisation of cancer services, I have also recently conducted research into the role of personal tutors in supporting students. Publications include the book *The Challenge of Person-centred Care: An Interprofessional Perspective* (2009) co-edited with Georgina Koubel.

Bob Cecil, Principal Lecturer in Social Work at Canterbury Christ Church University. I have a strong interest in interprofessionalism and also act as a consultant and trainer to a number of health and social care organisations. I am currently studying for a Doctorate in Education and have research interests in relation to theory and practice, transcultural practice and developing effective teaching and learning strategies for early stage learners. Prior to moving into social work education, I worked for many years in the areas of substance misuse and mental health.

Hazel Colyer, Senior Manager and Dean of Health and Social Care. My background is Therapeutic Radiography. I am active in professional role development and co-author of a number of reports about the scope of radiographic practice and the role of radiographers in cancer care services. I became involved in interprofessional education (IPE) in the early 1990s, initially as Programme Director of MSc and subsequently as Faculty Director of IPE. This role involved leading the development of undergraduate and postgraduate IPL Programmes. I have undertaken research in the area of IPL and competency and am active in the IPE Special Interest Group of the HEA Centre for Health Sciences and Practice.

Peter Ellis, MA Health Care Ethics, MSc Medical Epidemiology, BSc (Hons) Adult Nursing. I am a registered nurse with several years experience in renal nursing, research and management. Currently senior lecturer (Nursing) with expertise in research, public health, renal care, management and ethics, I have over 40 journal publications and have contributed to numerous books as well as editing and writing academic books. I have a special interest in the philosophical basis of rights and how these might function in health and social care and society at large.

Jane Greaves, MSc Health Promotion and Health Education. Currently Programme Director Specialist Community Public Health Nursing and Module Lead for the Practice Teacher Award. Following qualifying as a general nurse in Sydney Australia, I travelled to the United Kingdom to work, travel and study to be a midwife. It was during this experience that I was introduced to the field of health visiting, a career pathway that I was to eventually follow. Returning to Australia I was privileged to work as a midwife in the Northern Territory and this led to my resolve to understand further the public health dimension of children and families. Qualifying as a Health Visitor in Kent I have worked across several diverse communities in East Kent. My interest in interprofessional education and learning developed from working in Primary Care Trusts and the Kent, Surrey and Sussex GP and have developed this further by developing interprofessional working and learning between social workers, school nurses and health visitors. I have an interest in the support of those living in marginalised communities, health inequalities and supporting practice teachers.

Georgina Koubel, MSc Interprofessional Health and Community Studies, currently a senior lecturer in social work. Following several years undertaking generic social work in London, I moved to Kent where I have specialised in developing my interest in the area of Adult Services. In addition to working as a care manager, I have been a practice teacher, and an Adult Services training manager/consultant, developing new training programmes for practitioners in Kent Adult Social Services. Since taking up the role of senior lecturer (social work) in 2003, I have built on my experience within interprofessional education, currently taking on the lead for the Post Qualifying Specialist Social Work pathway for practitioners in Adult Services. I have particular interests and expertise in the areas of adult safeguarding, equalities and diversity, disability discourses and person-centred approaches to working with vulnerable adults and their networks.

Janet Melville-Wiseman, DipSW, CQSW, Cert in Psychotherapy, MSc, PhD Principal Lecturer in Social Work and Professional Lead for Social Work. I have many years experience of working as a social work practitioner, manager and academic. My interests include mental health social work with adults and older people, social inequalities, gender, ethics and conceptualisations of risk. I am also interested in developing the usefulness of case study as a method in social work research. Areas of research have included understanding the needs of older people in rural areas, evaluating regulation of social care and responses to professional sexual abuse in the mental health system

Andy Nazarjuk, senior lecturer in learning disability. My background is in community health care nursing and I began my teaching career as a lecturer practitioner in the early 1990s. My experience of interprofessional education has developed over a number of years being involved in pre- and post-registration interprofessional programmes. My specialist subject area is learning disability nursing which enables me to teach students from a range of specialities and I am currently module leader for a core module, interprofessional collaboration and person-centred care, within our continuing professional development framework. My key areas of interest are the history and marginalisation of people with a learning disability, disability issues, inclusion and the use of imagery and film in teaching.

Cheryl Yardley, MSc Applied Social Studies (Oxon). My practice background is in social work with children and families, in child protection and family support for a local authority and for a Sure Start programme. Since joining the university in 2006, I have taken on responsibility for the Post Qualifying Specialist Social Work Framework, developing the current programme and taking the lead for the Children and Families pathway. My particular areas of interest are Safeguarding Children, child development, the assessment of risk, and domestic violence, and I have carried out research into domestic violence perpetrated by young people against their parents.

Introduction

Georgina Koubel and Hilary Bungay

The motivation and inspiration for writing this book came from working with undergraduate and post-qualifying students in health and social work. Over many years, it has become apparent that the situations in practice that give people the most stress and cause the most tension and anxiety are those that involve the struggle to achieve an acceptable balance between often conflicting rights and risks when engaging with service users. In many situations, particularly those involving levels of risk to vulnerable people who use services, the expectations of the press and the public may be seriously at odds with the requirements of the employer and these may further conflict with the professional ethics and values of the practitioner concerned.

Although complex issues in health and social care nearly always demand collaborative interprofessional working, there may on occasions also be areas of disagreement among professionals from diverse agencies. Sometimes these are relatively easy to resolve but at other times it may be difficult to understand the lack of communication and cooperation. Throughout the book there is an emphasis on 'surfacing' and trying to understand different models and approaches, on the basis that if we can understand the source of the views of other professionals, there is a better chance that we can value each others' perspectives and work more effectively together. The most important aspect of this is that it should then improve communication among professionals, build better relationships with service users and provide a better, more coherent and therefore if necessary more supportive response in situations of risk and uncertainty.

A good example of this is that there may be different ways of understanding how we construct and make sense of the notion of vulnerability. A purely medical model may assume that an adult is vulnerable because they are ill, or of a certain age, or because they have a physical or learning disability. In some ways this has been the model that society has accepted for so long that it feels almost like common sense. But social analysts of disability, many of whom are people who themselves have experienced impairment, find that a social model of disability is more appropriate to their sense of who they are.

Taking this as a framework, Martin (2007) discusses a social model of vulnerability where it is the lack of adaptation in the environment and the attitudes of others that make people vulnerable rather than the inherent impairments. Attitudes which limit people's rights and expectations and which make assumptions about what people with disabilities cannot do, rather than supporting them to achieve their own goals and dreams can be far more disabling than the level of impairment. Most significantly, a social model constructs disabled people as citizens within society with the same rights as any other citizen. However, this sense of rights is accompanied by a reciprocal sense of responsibilities and the balance between these two is part of the analysis that will be taking place throughout this book.

For practitioners within health and social care and those who are seeking to join them, risk appears to be a key feature of the work of those who are involved in practice with vulnerable people. Whether working with children or vulnerable adults, practitioners need to be aware of the models and values they bring to their work, and the impact this can have on work with people who are facing areas of risk in their lives.

It is not only the construction of vulnerability that differs between the disciplines, but also the language used to refer to people accessing services, and indeed health and social care students. For example, throughout the book different professions use 'patients', 'service users' or 'clients' to describe the people with whom they interact. Similarly when the authors of different chapters refer to the students within their disciplines they use 'pre-registration' or 'pre-qualifying' depending on whether they are referring to health or social care students. Where social workers or health practitioners are undertaking further study they are referred to as 'post-qualifying' or 'post-registration' to distinguish them from undergraduates. Whilst language can be a barrier to effective interprofessional collaborative working recognising the existence and meaning of profession specific jargon and the value base which supports it can overcome the difficulties of understanding each other's perspectives. In a person-centred approach to care it is preferable to avoid labels and jargon but in practice they are in common usage and therefore the book reflects the reality of everyday life.

However, one of the strengths of this book is that it is not only written by a range of health and social care professionals including: an adult nurse, community nurse, mental health and learning disability nurses, public health nurse, radiographers (diagnostic and therapeutic), social workers (adult services and children and family services), but also members of different disciplines have co-written a number of the chapters. As a result, the perspectives of health care practitioners in the acute sector where the medical model of care predominates, and the perspectives of health and social care practitioners working in the community where the social model of care is central are integrated to provide a collaborative approach to rights, risks and responsibilities.

When assessing risk the medical approach generally is to look at the rational or scientific factors and the odds of an adverse event occurring, whereas the social approach looks at other influences and uses a number of different models to assess risk and assist decision making. Throughout this book all people are assumed to be potentially vulnerable at different stages of their life course. It is apparent whichever approach to risk assessment is adopted the rights and responsibilities surrounding the care of vulnerable people must be taken into account.

The book is presented in two main parts, Part I provides an introduction to the 'Theoretical Concepts and Constructs' around responsibilities, rights and risk. In Part II, 'Theory in Practice', each chapter uses specific areas of practice to demonstrate how theory can be applied. In each chapter we have also included case studies and reflective exercises that we have called *challenges*, these have been written to help you to reflect on the issues raised, and to explore your own attitudes and experiences surrounding rights, risks and responsibilities.

In the first chapter Ellis defines rights and responsibilities and how they function at an individual level and as a basis for relationships between providers and recipients of health and social care. Ellis uses a number of case studies to help the reader explore what rights and responsibilities mean both for the professional and as an individual. One of the case studies relates the notion of citizenship and explores how this may have an influence on the right of the individual to care in the United Kingdom. In a further case study some of the issues that occur when considering the concept of 'duty of care' in health and social care provision are identified. Throughout the chapter Ellis considers the ethical dimensions of care, including the right to care, the nature of human interests, and the tensions that may arise for practitioners when considering the best interests of an individual. The reader is challenged to question their assumptions about rights and how they apply to the services health and social care professionals deliver.

Following this, in Chapter 2 Bungay uses the examples of medical screening and vaccination to assist the understanding of risk and how people balance risks and benefits when making decisions around health and well-being. As Adams in Chapter 3 describes, there is currently emphasis on the individual to take responsibility for their own health. Citizens of the UK are entitled to access a range of health promoting, and illness preventing services offered by the National Health Service (NHS), including screening, childhood vaccinations and information regarding diet, exercise smoking and alcohol consumption. Despite these services being free, uptake is rarely 100 per cent as people choose not to attend. Bungay explores how risk is communicated to the general public and how this may influence risk assessment, and also the rights of the individual to make choices regarding lifestyles and where responsibility lies for maintaining healthy lives. In addition to exploring choices that otherwise healthy people make Bungay uses a case study to explore the rights of vulnerable people to access health promotion services and the issues that may arise in balancing risks and rights.

In Chapter 3 Adams introduces the notion that an increased awareness of 'risk' has shaped our experience of society, and that successive governments' responses to risk and their beliefs as to where responsibility for managing risk lies, has impacted upon the provision of health and social care services. He considers the relationship between individuals and the state providing an examination of the rights, risks and responsibilities in the political and historical context. Arguing that civic and human rights and responsibilities originate from the concept of citizenship, Adams demonstrates how the shifts in ideology over the past century have resulted in a move away from the notion of individual responsibility for welfare to that of collective responsibility, followed by the role of the state being reduced and the onus being placed back on the individual in more recent years. This shift has taken place in conjunction with a heightened perception of risk in everyday life and the shift in responsibility so too has led to the assessment of risk being left to the individual to manage their own fate. Adams concludes that in an uncertain world there are complex and powerful forces that shape societies and our own responses to rights, risks and responsibilities.

Koubel and Yardley in Chapter 4 look at different models of risk assessment and risk management and how these can be applied to complex situations involving vulnerable people. The authors are both social workers; one with experience with children and families and the other in adult services. Koubel and Yardley use two case studies to illustrate the use of these models; one involving a child in a family, and the other a disabled person living in the community. Each case raises issues of risk, safeguarding and protection and explores the balance of rights, choice and capacity, and legal and ethical frameworks are used to inform their analysis. The authors outline the potential risks within each situation and then apply different methods of risk assessment to demonstrate how some models of risk assessment may lead to a more flexible and less risk adverse approach to risk. The purpose of this is to enable the practitioner to consider a wider range of factors and potential outcomes and in particular focusing on actions which may reduce risk. Although this chapter's focus is on scenarios that may occur in the community and involve social workers, the different models of risk assessment presented could also be usefully applied within the health care sector.

There are a number of complexities surrounding the rights, risks and responsibilities of profoundly disabled individuals. Nazarjuk and Bernal in Chapter 5 start by identifying what is meant by the term 'profound intellectual and multiple disabilities' (PIMD) and then describe the historical development of the care for people with PIMD and how this has contributed to the continuing exclusion of this group by society. People with PIMD are an exceptionally vulnerable group of people and the authors consider the factors which contribute to this vulnerability, and the abuse they may experience (institutional, psychological and sexual) as a result. A number of case studies are used to help the reader explore and understand the rights of people with PIMD, and the responsibilities of those that care. Nazarjuk and Bernal conclude by discussing approaches that may promote the rights of people with PIMD such as improved communication by people working with them and person-centred active support.

Practitioners working in health and social care may come into contact with people who misuse substances; such people are sometimes labelled as drug addicts and alcoholics, and are stereotyped and stigmatised by society. In Chapter 6 Cecil provides an introduction to the key concepts surrounding substance misuse and explores ways in which practitioners can develop a more informed approach to their assessment of risk and decision making when working with this group of people. As with other chapters in this book Cecil uses practice based vignettes to illustrate particular discussion points, and by the end of the chapter non-specialists should have a greater awareness of the key ethical debates around different approaches to dealing with problem drinking, the misuse of drugs and other substances.

People within the mental health services, like all individuals, have relationships with family, friends and the community in which they live. They also have a relationship with the professionals and practitioners who have responsibility for their care. In Chapter 7, Melville-Wiseman considers the different aspects of relational risks, rights and responsibilities that practitioners may experience when working with people with mental health needs. She also explores the complex range of issues relating to the assessment of relational needs in risk management. There is discussion around the inequalities in relationships and how to keep relationships in mental health services safe. The overall focus of the chapter is on the importance of understanding past experiences of relational violence and abuse, particularly for women with mental health needs and the potential impact on their future relationships.

In Chapter 8, Greaves and Yardley consider the professional roles and responsibilities in managing risk and safeguarding children. Coming from different professional backgrounds; a social worker and a public health nurse, they use their experiences of interprofessional working and learning to inform their discussion on the different professional perspectives and how these can impact on decision making and the assessment of risk. A key message throughout the chapter is the need for professionals to work together to improve the quality of care and outcomes for service users. They conclude that interprofessional learning is essential to enable a greater understanding of each other's roles and responsibilities, and can help to overcome preconceived assumptions about levels of knowledge and the stereotyping that occurs, and which may hinder effective communications and thus the safeguarding of vulnerable children.

Koubel and Arnott, a social worker and a community nurse, in Chapter 9 together explore health and social care in the community and the issues surrounding risks, rights and responsibilities in relation to working with older people in the community setting. With the aim of fostering collaborative working between different professionals they look at a number of areas including the medical and social models of risk, perceptions of professional accountability and ageist attitudes to vulnerability. They acknowledge that there is the potential for conflict and tensions in complex situations involving one or more service users, their families and the wider community. They highlight the need to consider the rights of the autonomous person to choose to take risks, and the issue of professional responsibilities where the person is incapacitated or vulnerable and unable to take decisions for themselves.

Throughout the book professional decision making and the differential responsibilities of practitioners involved in health and social care have been explored in relation to rights and risks. In Chapter 10 Colyer uses the example of cancer care to look at the sources of professional decision making and the influence of values and cultures. There is also an exploration of the communication barriers that exist within teams and how this can affect the outcomes for the patient. She acknowledges that there is the potential for collaborative working to fail if members of the interprofessional team do not recognise the others' autonomy. Effective team working requires trust and for decision making to be transparent and accepted as legitimate by the team. Colyer concludes by asking readers to reflect on their own practice and how to balance professional accountability with collaborative working and the strategies that may be utilised to overcome the barriers to effective team working.

In Chapter 11 Koubel explores a number of themes emerging from the previous chapters, paying particular attention to how models of disability and vulnerability can affect the ways in which practitioners respond to the dilemmas which may emerge in relation to the rights and risks of service users and their carers and networks. She asks the reader to examine their own attitudes to risk and to think about the application and limits of particular models of risk assessment. She further highlights the importance of valuing the strengths, views and perspectives of all stakeholders involved in situations, and the challenge of ensuring the service user's voice is heard.

A reflective, integrated model, addressing knowledge, skills and values that would be expected to inform good practice in health and social care, is presented for the reader to enhance the development of a thoughtful, informed and measured approach to complex practice. Insights from the case study are then integrated to show how this model can relate to the analysis of rights, risks and responsibilities.

The Conclusion looks to the uncertain future of health and social care and highlights uncertainty about the changes that may be coming in relation to practice with children and adults who may be at risk. At present it is unclear whether the changes will result in more restrictive forms of intervention or whether vulnerable people will be left to manage their own lives with less help (or interference) than previously. Either way there will be considerable challenges for those employed within the health and social care workforce. The Conclusion reiterates the need for conscientious practitioners to reflect carefully on their values and practice, and to find ways to work closely with each other and to engage appropriately with service users to manage the delicate blend of rights, risks and responsibilities.

Reference

Martin, J. (2007) *Safeguarding Adults*. Lyme Regis: Russell House.

PART

I

Theoretical Concepts and Constructs

Rights and Responsibilities

Peter Ellis

Introduction

This chapter aims to define what rights and responsibilities are and how they function both at a human level and as the basis for the relationships we have with our
patients and clients within the caring professions. Within the chapter a philosophical and legal/contractual basis for the creation, meaning, purpose and operation
of rights and what these might indicate in terms of professional responsibilities
will be examined and applied to scenarios which occur in care provision. The
concept of best interests as a moral reason for the creation of rights will be
explored to see if they can provide some form of answer to the questions about
the purpose of rights and what these mean in relation to the duty of care.

Throughout the chapter the reader is challenged to question their own
assumptions about what rights are, what purpose they serve and how they
might be put into action within health and social care practice.

LEARNING OUTCOMES

By the end of the chapter you should have developed your understanding
of:

- What rights and responsibilities mean for you as a professional and
  human being

- The basis of special rights and responsibilities and the nature of the
  'duty of care'

➜

➜

- What it might mean to have interests as a human being

- How these interests might translate into rights and corresponding responsibilities.

The purpose of rights and responsibilities

The philosophical, political and legal basis of rights and responsibilities as they apply to life in general as well as to care provision needs to be understood and accepted by health and social care professionals in order to inform their activities. Many of the ethical and moral challenges which face health and social care practitioners in the twenty-first century can be better laid bare, and subsequently understood, if those same professionals have a working understanding of the basis of human rights and what these mean in relation to being a citizen as well as a caring professional. Without such an understanding of what rights and responsibilities are the adoption of professional values has a limited cognitive, philosophical and practical basis.

Vulnerability is both a reality and a social construct and many of the people we care for are vulnerable either because of a specific situation they find themselves in, for example following a trauma, or more generally because they have a long-term condition or are considered to be disabled.

With regard to protecting those who are vulnerable the nature and purpose of rights within this context are twofold; the first is they protect the individual from unwarranted and unwanted interference from others and, second they create a situation whereby others have a responsibility, or duty, to help. This creates some interesting scenarios for the operation of rights in the care setting where the individual who has a right:

- may choose not to use it;

- may choose to use it in what the care professionals regard as a counter-intuitive way;

- may not even know they have it;

- has it protected by the care professionals even when they do not want this or

- has it ignored by the professionals.

Throughout the chapter several of these scenarios will be explored in the form of real and imaginary case studies; you may do well to think of cases that you have been involved in for yourself and use the theory presented here to work through the ethical issues they throw up.

It is worth remembering at this stage that there are other approaches to the ethics of care which may be used to inform our decision making with clients.

Such approaches include the now rightly famous four principles plus scope approach presented by Beauchamp and Childress (2008): respect for autonomy, beneficence (doing good), nonmaleficence (avoiding harm) and justice. This rule-based approach provides an insight into the areas of both values and action which might inform our day-to-day decision making in the health and social care setting. While the leading competitor approach to ethics, consequentialism suggests that the ends justify the means.

Clearly any ethics of care has to take into account the supremacy of the individual; in rule-based approaches this is by paying regard over and above all else to the autonomy of the individual, while in consequentialism this is seen in the nature of the outcome of an intervention which may be regarded as good because it protects something important, like autonomy, or promotes justice.

This chapter will, however, concentrate on rights which are generally poorly understood, but when employed judiciously allow care professionals not only to protect those we serve, but also allow us to exercise some of the values which are central to our identity; things like protecting autonomy, social justice, doing the right thing, not doing harm and achieving the right ends.

What rights are

What rights are and what they serve to do is perhaps not as easy a question to answer as it might first appear. Rights exist for a number of reasons and to do a number of important jobs. For the purposes of this chapter, and indeed the book, rights might best be thought of as operating at two distinct levels: the human (also called natural) and the legal or contractual level. Interestingly these two levels are not always distinct one from the other. The Human Rights Act 1998 (HRA) which came into force in UK law in October 2000, giving effect to the European Convention for the Protection of Human Rights and Fundamental Freedoms (Council of Europe, 1950) appears to transcend both interpretations. On the one hand, it seeks to defend rights which perhaps exist purely by virtue of the fact that they protect peoples' natural rights, while on the other hand the HRA exists to both create and defend people's legal rights. (See Table 1.1 for an outline of the key elements of the HRA and what they might mean for people working in health and social care.)

Hart (1992) defines having a right as having a moral justification for limiting how others act. Different rights theorists, however, mean different things when they say *x* has a right to *y*. Most of the definitions of what it might mean to have a right are captured in the following classic definitions by Hohfeld (1919, cited in Waldron 1992):

1. A liberty right means one has at the very least no duty to anyone not to do something
2. A claim right means that one has a claim that others will not interfere with you doing something (a negative claim) or a claim that others will help you achieve something (a positive claim)

3. A power, which is essentially the ability to change the form of a right that one has; e.g. releasing someone from an obligation
4. Immunity, where no-one can change the character of the right that one possesses.

This may at first glance appear quite confusing; however, there is a certain necessity to understand the purpose, and operation, of rights in order to inform the debates that occur day to day in health and social care practice during which people evoke rights, duties and the like. For instance, if a patient or client is to evoke a right in relation to the care that they are to receive it is important to understand what this right requires of us by the way of action or non-interference.

Within each of the above definitions of a right there are three separate elements: the right holder; the nature of the right and what the right requires of others. Understanding how these elements operate and interact will help us make sense of situations where rights are raised.

CHALLENGE

Within your own practice setting consider how the different definitions of rights discussed above might be seen to operate. What examples can you give of clients having a liberty, claim, power or immunity right? Who held the right, what did the right mean and what did it require of other people?

Within the UK system of health and social care provision, citizens are at liberty to access health and social care services provided by the National Health Service (NHS) and social services. They also have a strong positive claim right to care under the contractual agreement individuals (discussed later in the chapter) enter into when joining the caring professions and accept the corresponding 'duty of care'. So the right holder is the citizen, the nature of the right is a claim right to care and what is required of care professionals is that they provide this care (the so-called 'duty of care').

What is not always clear is the nature and scope of this care we are obliged to provide. Competing claims and finite resources create potential dilemmas in meeting the demands of care provision. Questions arise about what care should be provided and under what circumstances and indeed about who is entitled to receive that care (a positive claim right). Organisations such as the National Institute for Health and Clinical Excellence and the Social Care Institute for Excellence attempt to answer these questions through the provision of national guidelines which in essence determine what care people have the right to expect. Regardless of the availability of national guidelines there remain frequent, heated public debates about what the scope of care should be and, hence, what care people have the right to expect is provided for them.

Conversely, but not divorced from the debate about what rights to care citizens should have are the debates about what society should fund in the way of care. Consider the following case studies.

Table 1.1 The key elements of the Human Rights Act 1998 and what they might mean for care providers

Right	Why this is important in health and social care
Article 2 – Right to life.	Establishes the liberty right of individuals to be allowed to live their life in a manner they see fit while respecting the rights of others. This right recognises the ethical concept of the 'sanctity of life'.
Article 3 – 'No-one shall be subjected to torture or inhuman or degrading treatment or punishment' – unqualified right.	This establishes benchmarks against which to measure the quality of care and the way in which it is provided. It underpins the concept of dignity in care. This right also serves to remind care providers of the duty to avoid harm.
Article 5 – Right to liberty and security of the person – subject to exceptions, for example lawful detention after conviction, lawful arrest or detention to bring someone suspected of committing an offence to court, lawful detention to prevent the spread of disease, lawful detention of 'persons of unsound mind', alcoholics, drug addicts or vagrants, lawful detention of a minor for the purposes of 'educational supervision' or to bring him before a court.	Clearly health and social care professionals have no right to interfere in the lives of others except where the individual chooses for them to do so or where the individual is a risk to him/herself or others. The caveats here establish the reasonableness of detaining individuals who are incapable of making such choices for themselves. Where the exceptions do not operate, then care professionals are reminded of the need to respect autonomy.
Article 8 – Everyone has the right to respect for his private and family life, his home and his correspondence. There shall be no interference by a public authority with the exercise of this right except such as is in accordance with the law and is necessary in a democratic society in the interests of national security, public safety or the economic well-being of the country, for the prevention of disorder or crime, for the protection of health or morals, or for the protection of the rights and freedoms of others.	Here we are reminded that the people we care for exist in the context of their own lives, families and communities. The need to recognise, respond to and support the rights of the individual to be the person that they wish to be within this context is clearly identified. To a great extent this right serves to remind us of the importance of person-centred care, rather than provider driven care. Our duty here is that of justice – treating each person fairly.
Article 9 – Freedom of thought, conscience and religion.	Prompts care professionals to be mindful of the autonomy of individuals in choosing ways of life which are commensurate with their beliefs but which may conflict with what we regard as being in their 'best interests'; there is more to being human than mere physical functioning.
Article 14 – The enjoyment of the rights and freedoms set forth in this Convention shall be secured without discrimination on any ground such as sex, race, colour, language, religion, political or other opinion, national or social origin, association with a national minority, property, birth or other status.	Recognises that the primary moral criteria driving care provision is being human. Race, gender, age and the like are not morally relevant and should not impact on the way in which care is provided. This serves to protect equity, treating people fairly, and in relation to criteria which are morally relevant.

CASE STUDY

Joe is a 60-year-old man who is in need of a hip replacement. Joe is clinically obese weighing some 120 kg while being only five feet six inches tall. The orthopaedic surgeon says to Joe that despite his otherwise good health he will not operate on him because he does not believe in operating on people who are very obese. He says to Joe that he has no right to expect the NHS to replace his hip when, at least in part, his excess weight has contributed to his mobility problems.

Vijay is 65 and a lifelong smoker. He has intermittent claudication in his lower legs and needs vascular surgery to relieve his pain. Vijay's surgeon agrees to do the procedure and advises him to stop smoking.

Jane is a keen amateur climber. On a recent expedition she damaged the cartilage in her knee which needs arthroscopy and subsequent surgery. Jane's orthopaedic surgeon is happy just to get on with the procedure as she is young and fit.

CHALLENGE

- What are the morally relevant criteria in operation in each of these scenarios?
- Which of these conditions is not related to a lifestyle choice?
- What are the rights of the people in these scenarios?
- Should any of them be treated in a manner different to the others?

These scenarios illustrate some interesting points about what some people might regard as deserving and less-deserving needs. Within each of these scenarios there is a right to care, although the interpretation of the right to care appears to be somewhat different despite the fact that in reality each of the scenarios might be said to derive from individual lifestyle choices. It could be argued that in the first scenario the surgeon does not want to operate on Joe because his surgery may be unsuccessful or the anaesthetic may endanger Joe's life, but this is not what is said to Joe. With Vijay there is some advice, but no conditions attached to the surgery and for Jane she is offered surgery with no issues being raised.

What these scenarios illustrate is the different ways in which the individual's right to care can be translated. Why this should be and whether it is morally defensible remain debatable.

Natural rights

The philosophical basis of natural, human rights is a complex area which has tested thinkers for millennia. Generally speaking natural rights are regarded as arising out of the moral criteria that all human beings possess them by virtue of being human, while legal and civil rights are the product of debate, subsequent legislation and contracts.

It is by no means certain that the understanding of rights will provide solutions to all of the ethical and moral issues that face us in practice. Some philosophers believe that rights form the basis of morality (Mackie 1992) while for others rights are an important component of political morality (Dworkin 1987) and for others still rights operate only as one of a number of moral and ethical precepts which might also include values, duties and utility (Raz 1992).

Natural rights were seen by some early theorists to derive from the will of 'God' or 'Nature' itself (Locke 1989). Thomas Hobbes, a seventeenth-century philosopher, was one of the first to articulate a theory of natural rights which reflects something of what we might understand within modern philosophy. His one natural right, which for him formed the basis of a social contract, was the right to self-preservation. This right arises out of the natural state and is carried through into societal living in order to protect two key human interests: to leave behind the natural state of human existence which was 'solitary, poore, nasty, brutish and short' (Hobbes 1991: 90) and the 'desire of such things that are necessary to commodious living' (Hobbes 1991: 90).

The message that Hobbes brings us here that is pertinent to health and social care provision today is that rights exist for specific reasons; they have a basis in something more important than themselves. So rights exist not only as entities in themselves, but to protect something that is regarded as significant. The right to life is a good example of this as life, in this sense, is seen as something that is worthy of the protection of a right. What constitutes life and what it might mean to have a right to life do, however, require some definition.

CHALLENGE

It is easy to consider that we know what is best for an individual in relation to their self-preservation and we readily form opinions about the choices that people make as being wise or unwise. Consider what self-preservation might mean to you not only in the physical, but also in the emotional, social and spiritual sense. Then consider how this might vary between different individuals because of their age, culture, religion or life experiences. Try discussing this with members of your family, friends, people at work or in the university.

What you may notice as a result of this challenge is that the things that you hold important and which essentially constitute the things that make you who you are, are in fact difficult to articulate – so how then can they be protected?

You might consider how you might feel if you were denied the opportunity to exercise the freedoms that allow you to live your life in a manner you regard as being good – and gain some understanding of what the 'self' in self-preservation means.

By understanding what is important to you, you may start to understand what is important to other people and thereby how you might protect those less able to exercise their human rights – although as our challenge demonstrates what is important to you may not be important to someone else.

It can be difficult for the health or social care professional to see past what they believe to be in the best interests of their clients. As caring professionals we often have a clear picture of what we would want for ourselves in a given situation as well as how we want to act when we are called upon to provide care.

The challenge here is to understand that what we may want for ourselves and what our clients may want for themselves may well be the same, but the ways in which we each wish to achieve the same ends may be very different (e.g. consider the very many different ideas about what dignity is). In these circumstances an understanding of the nature of rights enables us not only to ask the correct questions about the choices people make, but also to explore what the correct solutions to meeting conflicting rights may be. Simple dilemmas may appear in practice where a lonely widow with a mobility disability wants to use some of her direct payments to have her windows cleaned so she can look out on the world when you consider she should be using the money to buy personal care, or when a client with a learning disability uses her money to pay for a night out with her boyfriend even though her fridge is empty. In both cases what everyone wants is what is best for the client; the simple truth is in both scenarios what is best for the client is open to interpretation.

Interests as the basis of human rights

One way of helping us to understand what sort of ideas human rights might serve to protect is to explore issues around 'best interests'. The view that only beings that have interests can have moral rights is a view which has widespread appeal and support (Kuhse 1985; Ellis 1996). This does not necessarily mean that interests themselves are sufficient criteria for having rights, merely that those beings who have interests are the sort of beings on whom it is plausible to confer rights. From this view, rights may serve to protect some of the important interests people have and many of these important interests are what we see at work in care settings.

CHALLENGE

Stop for a moment and consider what might be meant by interests. What do you mean when you say 'it is in my best interests'? Does your definition of best interests appear to be something that deserves the protection of rights? You might like to have this discussion with colleagues at work or in the university setting. You will get most insight into this if you individually write down your ideas before sharing what you have written and discussing their meaning. Are the sorts of interests that operate in the social care setting different to those which affect health? Which interests are most important? Why?

Clearly not every definition of interests provides us with an answer as to what deserves the protection that rights confer – there is more to possessing rights than merely being a being capable of interests. What is needed is that the interests people have must be related to what philosophers term some 'human good'.

Regan (1976, cited in Kuhse 1985: 148) makes an important distinction between the two meanings of the term 'interest'; he says that 'Good health is in John's interests and John has an interest in good health'. In the first meaning 'interests' relate to John's well-being, in the second to a desire that John has. Certainly it is true that John both desires good health and that good health is good for him. What is not possible, nor perhaps morally desirable, is that we respect every desire that people have, since some desires may be wicked, misplaced or unachievable.

It is also true that some people we regard as having rights (e.g. people with dementia or those who are unconscious) may not even know, let alone be able to explain, what they want. It seems unlikely, therefore, that interests which relate to individual desires should have the protection of rights. What seems more reasonable is that rights should serve to defend those interests which relate to some aspect of an individual's well-being (good health is in John's interests); what, in translation, Aristotle would have called 'human flourishing' (Aristotle 1976).

CASE STUDY

Dave is a Jehovah's Witness who has been involved in a traumatic car crash. Dave is admitted to the emergency department with various injuries and has severe blood loss. In order to save Dave's life the team want to give him multiple blood transfusions, but Dave, who is still conscious, pleads with them not to do so as this is against his beliefs.

CHALLENGE

What might be meant by best interests in this scenario? Who defines best interests? Who should define best interests? Which definition of best interests deserves the protection of rights?

We can see from this case study that unlike John in the example from Regan, there are two conflicting views about what might be in the best interests of Dave. The medical and nursing team consider it to be in Dave's best interests for him to have a transfusion, while Dave, although perhaps realising that it is in his best interests medically does not see this as being in his personal best interest – which is a viewpoint recognised by the Department of Health (2001). The medical team may have a right to deliver good quality health care to Dave but this right conflicts with his right to make choices about how he lives his life and what is done to his body – what he considers to be his best interests.

There are clearly two forms of interest at work here. Dworkin (1993) usefully categorises these as 'experiential' and 'critical' interests. In the case of experiential interests Dworkin (1993) is referring to pleasurable or painful *experiences*. It is obvious that avoiding pain is in everyone's best interests, although what constitutes pain and pleasure may differ according to individual tastes and preferences. Critical interests, on the other hand, are the sort of interests that represent the things in life that we all need. Such critical interests represent the sorts of things that make life worthwhile and are more a matter of judgement than of taste. Dworkin (1993: 204) states that:

> We need an intellectual explanation of critical interests, so that we may better understand these ideas from the inside, understand introspectively how they connect with other large beliefs we have about life and death and why human life has intrinsic worth.

What critical interests are and why they deserve the protection of rights is hard to state precisely, but it would be fair to say that they are part of a shared human intuition about what is important in life.

Critical interests relate to the way that an individual chooses to lead their life and are believed by many philosophers to maintain their importance even if the individual to whom they pertain is unconscious or even dead (Feinberg, 1974) and whether or not they are capable of perceiving them as such (Veatch 1995). As Allmark *et al.* (2001: 122) note:

> An interest is something in which we have a stake, that is, we stand to lose or gain depending upon what happens to it. What is important here is that having an interest in something does not require being interested in it.

When thinking about the value of human life it is worth considering why as a society we tend to agree that gossiping about an individual is wrong even if they do not find out; why we say that one should not speak ill of the dead and why in the intensive care setting or theatres when people are unconscious we still talk to them and treat them with the same respect we would give them if they were aware.

Important critical interests that might deserve the protection of rights include maintaining a good reputation (Levenbook 1984), having respect, maintaining independence (Dworkin 1993), exercising autonomy, having meaningful relationships, accomplishing things and enjoying life (DeGrazia1995), as well as maintaining that elusive concept – dignity (Linacre Centre 1998).

There are some real tensions for the health or social care practitioner in considering these notions of best interests. For example, if the interest in maintaining independence is afforded the protection of rights, what are the corresponding duties of the social care team in enabling their client to achieve this? If such a right is afforded the status of a positive claim right as opposed to a liberty or negative claim right, where does the duty to provide this stop and who in society does this duty fall to?

CASE STUDY

Emily is a lady in her seventies who is struggling to live at home on her own. It is clear after a series of falls and other minor incidents that she would be 'better off' in residential care. Emily refuses to go into a home because she wants to maintain as much of her independence as possible. The cost of providing intensive social care to her at home is increasing as her needs escalate and have reached a point where residential care is now more financially viable and probably safer.

It is easy to forget among the economic factors and 'common sense' approach to care that basic human needs are often the issues that cause patients the most distress. In the case study above, Emily clearly has a right to have her wishes to live as independently as possible respected. This scenario is not only about an elderly lady wishing to remain at home, it is about respecting Emily's interest in maintaining her reputation and independence – her dignity if you like. As has been argued above, such interests may well deserve the protection of rights.

So if Emily has a right to have her interest in maintaining her dignity protected, what does this mean for the social care team looking after her? Certainly on a human level there is no direct duty on social services to help her fulfil these wishes, although there may be a duty for her not to interfere with Emily in the process of fulfilling them herself.

Surely if Emily had a positive claim right to have all of her care at home, as a human being then this right has to extend to all such persons? This simply cannot be the case as this would extend to the whole of humanity and we would all be encumbered with the need to support all those in a similar situation. Think about it this way: your neighbours, as fellow humans, have a right to be able to keep themselves clean and thereby protect their dignity, but because you have no relationship with them either in the family or care sense you are not under any obligation to help them achieve this.

Somehow this simple explanation, while following the line of argument to date, seems wrong both intuitively and as a caring professional. This is because human rights, *per se*, are not perhaps the best explanation for the basis of the 'duty of care' as we know it.

Legal/contractual rights

Understanding the duties we have towards our patients and clients as caring professionals requires that we look at other justifications of rights. It seems reasonable to presuppose as care professionals that the obligations we have to those we care for go beyond the obligations that exist in society as a whole.

Hart (1992) calls the sort of rights that exist in the care setting between the carer and the cared for 'special rights'. Special rights are the result of a transaction, or special relationship, between two parties; the sort of thing that arises from making a promise. So if Hannah promises to help Izzy with the school run, Izzy's right to expect Hannah to help arises purely from the fact Hannah has promised. The moral status of the promise arises out of the fact it is made voluntarily.

What then does this mean for the care professional? Surely we do not go around making promises to our patients all of the time and therefore enter into a morally relevant relationship? Think again, because in fact we probably do.

Special rights arise out of people consenting, authorising and submitting to mutual restrictions. Cooperation is the key to this genre of rights, with individuals expecting the submission of others to the same rules as apply to them. The obligations that arise are thus not due to the fact that those involved are human as such, rather it is because they agree to cooperate. In the care setting professionals agree to take on the mantle of caring for others in return for pay, so the rights thus created between caring professionals and those in need of care are contractual in nature.

The contractual nature of the duty of care that care professionals submit to arises, in the UK at least, out of the contract we have with society at large. We agree to provide care and society agrees to pay us and afford us some level of respect.

Because this sort of right arises out of contracts between people – in the case of the National Health and social services between all citizens of the UK – the right to NHS provided health care and social care only extends to those people who meet the criteria of citizenship (see Adams, Chapter 3 for clarification of the concept of citizenship). This may seem harsh, but remember this is about the special, contractual right to *health care* and not the universal liberty right to *health* that might arise from a consideration of interests and human rights.

CASE STUDY

Reg has arrived in the UK illegally. He has travelled to the UK from the Cameroon in order to seek medical care for his rapidly advancing liver failure which was caused by hepatitis C. Reg is admitted to the liver intensive care unit in need of a liver transplant in order to stay alive. Reg is a teacher and has a large family for whom he is the main bread winner.

Dorothy, a UK citizen, has alcoholic liver disease, she is a retired secretary who lives alone and has no living relatives. Like Reg, Dorothy needs a liver transplant to stay alive.

Ben is a university student in his early twenties who was born with liver disease; he also needs a transplant to transform his life.

Reg, Dorothy and Ben share the same blood group and would be eligible for the same liver when one becomes available. Who has the strongest right to receiving a liver? Why?

This sort of scenario is always emotive. There would appear to be a strong humanitarian motivation for transplanting all of these individuals. It might be argued by some that Dorothy was less deserving than the other two as she had a disease which was self-inflicted; Reg may appear to some not to be eligible because he has not contributed to the NHS through national insurance; while Ben, who also has made no contributions, might arguably be the most deserving as he is a UK citizen and is not responsible for his disease and has the most to gain in terms of quality adjusted life years.

Clearly following the themes of the chapter, each of these individuals has a right to life which having the transplant might fulfil. The right to life may be justifiable as a human right, but only in so far as it is a liberty right; which would translate to something like: no-one should take someone else's life without just cause. This clearly means that no-one is under any obligation to save the life of any of these three individuals.

Regardless of the blame attached to the disease, each of the people within this scenario does have an absolute human right to have their dignity respected – this being a fundamental human interest. Having one's dignity respected is not the same, however, having a claim to having a life-saving operation. From the point of view of the special rights that accrue through citizenship, only Dorothy and Ben might be said to have any claim to the liver transplant and subsequent care.

The difficulty lies in the fact that both claims to the liver cannot be honoured and therefore the strengths of the competing rights must be considered along with other morally relevant criteria. Among these are notions of the duty of care of the health care professionals involved; which most certainly extend beyond only considering the well-being of those immediately in front of them.

The duty of care

We have so far identified some bases on which rights to care might be founded. What we have not examined is what one person's right means for others. Some commentators argue that rights are difficult to deal with moral concepts because they always create a corresponding duty on the part of others and this creates an undue burden. This view is at least in part correct, but what constitutes a duty and what this requires in the way of action need to be defined.

Philosophically not all duties arise from considerations of rights. Certainly deontologists, such as the famous Immanuel Kant, believe in a scheme of ethical duties by which people are bound because they support the notion that all people are in fact ends in themselves, rather than means to an end (Kant 1991). Such duty-based ethical theorists maintain human actions are right or wrong in themselves regardless of the consequences of the action and according to reason we all have an obligation to act in ways which these duties prescribe – these duties are created through rational reflection which leads to self-evident truths.

The guiding principles of this school of thought include the notions of autonomy and freedom of action. Kant (1991: 51) argues that the universal categorical imperative that applies to the formulation and action of any duty is that we should only 'act upon a maxim that can also hold as a universal law'. That is, only act in such a way you would be happy for others to act in relation to you.

While deontology has much to offer in relation to insights into how and why we should treat others fairly, it is perhaps reasonable to say any duties relating to the provision of care cannot be subsumed within this ethical scheme because of their extensive, universal, scope. Such universal duties to provide health and social care create scenarios where no-one's care needs would be met properly.

━━━━━━━━━━━━━━━━━━━━━━━ **CHALLENGE** ━━━━━━━━━━━━━━━━━━━━━━━

What might be the consequences for care provision if we were to accept that everyone had the same natural positive claim rights to total health and social care provision, rather than a liberty right to health *per se*? What would this mean for the provision of health and social care provision and for humanity in trying to provide this health care?

━━

From the arguments made thus far, there are some clear natural or human rights which are afforded to all by virtue of their humanity. Evidently the ideals that such rights serve to protect are fundamental to the existence of society. Ethics, as a discipline, and as a guide to action, is a response to the fact that we, as humans, live in societies. The problem with accepting that all of us, and perhaps caring professionals in particular, have an absolute positive duty of care to all humanity has been mentioned already. If we accepted a positive claim right for all humanity to health and social care then we would all be obliged, by duty, to provide this care. This is simply unrealistic. As fellow humans we may have absolute obligations not to harm the health or welfare of others and we may choose to provide care to those to whom we are not obliged, but this is perhaps the tenable limit of this broader obligation; the lack of an overriding duty of care makes all acts of kindness to those we are not obliged to help all the more laudable.

The obligations to provide care that apply to members of the caring professions arise out of the rights of members of society. As argued before, we accept an obligation, duty, to care when we *voluntarily* enter into the caring professions.

There are occasions when we have a right to withdraw from a care episode because we have some conscientious or religious objection to what is being done; an obvious example of this is the right not to be involved in the commission of surgical abortion. This right not to be involved in abortion does not extend to a right not to be involved in the care of the individual who has had the abortion for good reason. The right not to be involved in the commission of abortion is about the act of abortion itself; it is not a judgement about the individual, their morals or their status as a patient or client. As care professionals we have a right to object to the act and not the person *per se*.

This approach is reflected in the way that many parents say to their *naughty* children: 'I love you, but I do not like the way you are behaving!' Clearly in

both scenarios we still have a duty of care which is begot from the special relationship we have with the woman (as a care professional) or the child (as a
parent).

In society at large rights usually imply some obligation not to interfere with
the actions and activities of others so long as they are not interfering with us,
not acting illegally or are not harming themselves. The duty of care therefore
arises out of a special relationship but that relationship, like all relationships, has
to have realistic boundaries.

Conclusion

This chapter has identified and in part attempted to answer some of the questions that arise in relation to the idea of the duty of care in health and social
care provision. We have identified that the right to health care as it operates at
the moment in the UK is related to a special contract we enter into with each
other as a society in order to fulfil some basic human needs. We further identified that while there is most certainly a right to health which arises out of being
human, this right does not, however, create corresponding duties by which
others are bound.

We have examined the nature of human interests and how these might be
used to temper some of the more difficult debates we have about the detail of
the provision of health and social care within a system whereby the right to
health care has already been established. In part this argument is based on the
premise that ethics can only operate in a societal setting where the people who
make up the society accept there must be rules by which we all operate in order
to preserve the societal way of life. There is, and must, on the view discussed
within this chapter, however, be some pragmatic limits as to the duties that the
existence of rights impose upon us because without such limits societal living
would be impractical and that would be in no-one's best interests.

References

Allmark, P., Mason, S., Gill, A. B. and Megone, C. (2001) Is it in a neonate's best inter-
    est to enter a randomised controlled trial? *Journal of Medical Ethics*, 27: 110–13.
Aristotle (1976) *The Nicomachean Ethics* (trans. J. A. Thompson). London: Penguin.
Beauchamp, J. F. and Childress, T. L. (2008) *Principles of Biomedical Ethics* (6th edn).
    Oxford: Oxford University Press
Council of Europe (1950) European Convention for the Protection of Human Rights
    and Fundamental Freedoms. Available at: http://www.echr.coe.int/echr/en/
    header/the+court/events+at+the+court/60+years+of+the+convention (accessed 12
    October 2010).
Department of Health (2001) *Reference Guide to Consent for Examination or
    Treatment*. London: Department of Health.
DeGrazia, D. (1995) Value theory and the best interests standard. *Bioethics*, 9: 50–61.
Dworkin, R. (1987) *Taking Rights Seriously*. London: Duckworth.

Dworkin, R. (1993) *Life's Dominion: An Argument about Abortion and Euthanasia*. London: Harper Collins.

Ellis, P. (1996) Exploring the concept of acting in the patient's best interests. *British Journal of Nursing*, 5(17): 1072–4.

European Union (1998) The Human Rights Act. Available at: http://www.direct. gov.uk/en/Governmentcitizensandrights/Yourrightsandresponsibilities/DG_ 4002951 (accessed 12 October 2010).

Feinberg, J. (1974) The rights of animals and unborn generations. In W. Blackstone (ed.), *Philosophy and Environmental Crisis*. Georgia: University of Georgia Press.

Hart, H. L. A. (1992) Are there any Natural Rights? In J. Waldron (ed.), *Theories of Rights*. Oxford: Oxford University Press.

Hobbes, T. (1991) *Leviathan* (ed. R. Tuck). Cambridge: Cambridge University Press.

Kant, I. (1991) *The Metaphysics of Morals* (trans. M. Gregor). Cambridge: Cambridge University Press.

Kuhse, H. (1985) Words: Interests. *Journal of Medical Ethics*, 11: 146–9.

Levenbook, B. B. (1984) Harming someone after his death. *Ethics*, 94: 407–19.

Linacre Centre (1998) Human Dignity, Autonomy and Mentally Incapacitated Persons: A Response to *Who Decides?* Available at: http://www.linacre.org/whodec.html (accessed 29 October 2010).

Locke, J. (1989) *Two Treatises of Government* (ed. P. Laslett). Cambridge: Cambridge University Press.

Mackie, J. L. (1992) Can there be a rights based moral theory? In J. Waldron (ed.), *Theories of Rights*. Oxford: Oxford University Press.

Raz, J. (1992) Rights based moral theories. In J. Waldron (ed.), *Theories of Rights*. Oxford: Oxford University Press.

Veatch, R. M. (1995) Abandoning informed consent. *Hastings Centre Report*, 25: 5–12.

Waldron, J. (1992) Introduction. In J. Waldron (ed.), *Theories of Rights*. Oxford: Oxford University Press.

Rights, Risks and Healthy Choices

Hilary Bungay

Introduction

Decision making in health and social care often involves an assessment of risk, and the balancing of risk versus benefit. This chapter uses health screening and the vaccination programme to explore risk and the choices 'healthy' people make in relation to their health and well-being. Health is defined by the World Health Organisation (1946) as 'a state of complete physical, mental and social wellbeing, and not merely the absence of disease or infirmity'. This is a social model of health which adopts the perspective that the cause of ill health lies beyond pathological processes and recognises the influence of social and economic factors. The medical model on the other hand categorises disease on the basis of deviations from what is considered normal or the presence of a recognisable abnormality. The medical model is focused on the individual causes of ill health and emphasises disease and its prevention through targeting specific aetiologies, lifestyle choices, and the provision of interventions such as screening and vaccination.

Currently in England and Wales there is a range of health promoting strategies provided free at the point of delivery for the general population, including childhood vaccinations, flu jabs for older people, the national breast screening and cervical smear screening programmes. Such screening procedures are promoted as a means of diagnosing disease at an early stage, thus providing the chance of cure and reassurance for individuals, and vaccinations are given to prevent the transmission of potentially serious illnesses. Many would consider these to be highly desirable innovations yet the uptake of each of these screening and vaccinations programmes is rarely 100 per cent. When people are invited to these services each individual makes an assessment of the potential costs or risks of accepting the invitation and as part of this process the person has to weigh up the balance of risk against the predicted benefits. Yet public understandings and perceptions of risk are subjective and socially constructed how people perceive or measure their individual risk and whether they should or need to attend for screening or a vaccination is dependent on a number of influences, such as experience, level of anxiety, values, and increasingly the coverage in the media.

However, it is not only the perceived risk that will influence the uptake of these services but also the way in which the individual views responsibility for their own health and in the case of vaccination the health of their local community. Therefore the decision to attend for screening or vaccination is complex and for the lay person is rarely made purely on the basis of probability or statistics. Despite this when experts outline the risks and benefits of different procedures or interventions they commonly express the risk or probability of an adverse event happening in numerical terms such as 1 in 10 or 1 in 10,000 or use words such as negligible or moderate. Some people may not understand the implications of probability for them as individuals, and others are more risk adverse than others and vary in the levels of risk they are willing to accept in different circumstances. Whilst this chapter uses interventions in the health sector rather than social care to illustrate the factors which influence approaches to risk and the individual decision-making process, it is relevant to all health and social practitioners, as understanding how individuals may respond to perceived risk is essential when communicating with patients or service users to enable and empower people to make informed decisions about their care.

LEARNING OUTCOMES

By the end of the chapter you should have developed your understanding of:

- The scientific or rational approach to risk

- How to explain risk assessment in terms of statistics and probability

- How a person's assessment of risk is informed by cultural, social and lifestyle factors

- The process of balancing risk of a procedure/intervention or introduction of a care plan versus the potential for benefit

- The issues of trust and communication in relation to risk using the controversy of MMR vaccination as a case study.

The scientific or rational approach to risk

Risk is a word which when used generally refers to a threat rather than an opportunity, and on the whole refers to the possibility of something bad or undesirable occurring. So, for example, the weather forecaster may refer to the risk of heavy rain or snow but talk about the chance of sunshine and light showers. The meaning of risk is thought to derive from the Latin word *risco* used as a navigational term for sailors entering unchartered waters, and the Arabic word *risq* referring to the acquisition of wealth and good fortune (Skeat 1910, cited in Mythen 2004). The development of the statistical calculation of risk and probability had its origins in maritime insurance, and from a scientific perspective, risk is seen as the balance between threat and opportunity, and is measurable.

The majority of decisions taken in health and social care involve a risk assessment, such an assessment will depend upon identification or recognition of the hazard, an evaluation as to the potential seriousness of the hazard, and the probability of the hazard occurring (Greener 1996). It can be difficult for lay people to understand the probability of an event such as a side effect of a treatment occurring, but how such information is presented may well influence an individual's decision as to whether to go ahead with a therapeutic intervention such as taking a medicine or having surgery, or to attend for screening or vaccination.

Health and social care professionals play a key role in communicating information to the people for whom they care. As such they have a responsibility to convey relevant information in a form that is accessible and appropriate, and service users have the right to expect that the information that they are provided with is accurate to enable them to make an informed decision or choice about their care. Whilst consumers of health and social care services can supplement verbal information with information leaflets provided by government organisations which are hopefully reliable and evidence-based, there is also a multitude of web pages available on the internet some of which contain inaccuracies and inconsistencies. The language used in verbal or written sources may be technical and jargon-based and may therefore be inaccessible. There is therefore a potential imbalance in the level of knowledge between the lay person and professional which means that a degree of trust is required. Risk and trust are inextricably linked, and in recent times according to Beck (1999) accountability and responsibility have become part of the debates around risk, with the result that wherever a risk is perceived someone or some institution is held responsible for managing that risk, as we trust those in authority to protect us from harm. In health and social care the person (service-user or patient) needs to trust the professional to act in their best interests, and provide information appropriately (see Ellis, Chapter 1, for a discussion of best interests).

The rational approach to risk communication (Alaszewski 2005) emphasises the role and position of the experts as the guardians of the relevant knowledge, where this knowledge has been gained through education, research, experiential knowledge and is influenced by personal values. Levels of risk, and the probability of a hazard occurring (or not) can be communicated in a variety of ways, for instance the phrases 'minimal risk' or 'high risk' may be used, alternatively

Table 2.1 Explaining probability

Risk range (Numerical descriptors)	Probability of effect (EU 1998 verbal descriptors)	Level of risk Calman (1996)	Community Risk Scale (Calman and Royston 1997)
1 in a million 1:1,000000	Very rare	Negligible	The population of a large city e.g. Birmingham
Between 1 in a million and 1 in a hundred thousand 1:100,000–1:1,000000	Very rare	Minimal	
Between 1 in ten thousand and 1 in one hundred thousand 1:10,000–1:100,000	Very rare	Very low	The population of a large town e.g. Worthing (West Sussex)
Between 1 in a thousand to 1 in ten thousand 1:1000–1:10,000	Rare	Low	The population of a small town or the Isles of Scilly
Between 1 in a hundred to 1 in a thousand 1:100–1:1000	Uncommon	Moderate	A village
Greater than 1 in a hundred >1:100	Common	High	A street
1 in ten 1:10	Very common	Unknown risk – unquantifiable	A family

numbers or odds may be quoted, such as a 1 in 4 chance or one in a million. Table 2.1 demonstrates some of the ways that the probability of a risk occurring may be described or classified using Calman (1996), Knapp *et al.* (2004) and Calman and Royston (1997, in Department of Health 1997).

In column one (Table 2.1) the common numerical expressions or risk ratios (the odds) of an estimated risk that are used to define the frequency of a risk occurring is shown. However, such numbers can be misunderstood; if, for example, the ratios 1 in 25 and 1 in 200 are used some people may think that because 1:200 is the bigger number that it actually represents the greater risk.

To avoid such confusion Paling (2003: 746) suggests that when expressing odds that it is best practice to use a common denominator such as 40 out of 1000 and 5 out of 1000. In columns two and three the terms commonly used to describe or to relate approximate levels of probability are listed. In 1999 the European Union produced guidelines on the readability of leaflets included in medicine packs, it was suggested that the frequency of side effects could be denoted by the five verbal descriptors: very common, common, uncommon, rare, and very rare (Knapp *et al.* 2004). However, research has demonstrated that using verbal terms to describe the frequency or likelihood of an adverse event occurring are more likely to be misinterpreted by patients than numerical expressions, leading them to overestimate the probability of side effects occurring (Knapp *et al.* 2004), this is obviously undesirable if it means they then do not take the prescribed medication. The European Union descriptors define any event with a frequency of greater than 1 in 10,000 as being very rare. Calman (1996), on the other hand, also uses the words minimal and negligible, suggesting that a minimal risk is one that may be used in public policy to describe an 'acceptable' risk, and a negligible risk is one where there is a remote or insignificant chance of an adverse event occurring. Calman also states that some risks are unquantifiable because their extent is as yet unknown. This shows that there is not yet consensus between experts as to the best way of describing risks. Despite this, as Douglas (1992) points out, whilst experts assume that the general public are unable to understand the probabilities of risk, people have always made calculations about risk and the chance of adverse events occurring to them personally. As numerical phrases and words can be problematic because of the possible differing interpretations, alternative methods of explaining risk have been developed. For example, Paling (2003) suggested that to help overcome poor numeracy skills pictures or diagrams could be used to represent the numbers of those affected within populations, demonstrating the levels of risk visually. Another aid to understanding risk is the 'community risk scale' developed by Calman and Royston (Department of Health 1997: 10). This uses simple familiar comparisons such as 'about one person living in a small town', this concept has been developed in Table 2.1 (last column on the right) using data taken from the Office of National Statistics (2008) to provide real examples from communities in the United Kingdom to demonstrate the order of magnitude of risk. Therefore something that is described as having a risk of one in a million represents the risk of one person living in a city such as Birmingham of experiencing the adverse event, whereas a risk of one in a hundred corresponds to the risk to one person living in a street.

CHALLENGE

Could you think of another method of explaining the level of risk to a patient or service user?

It is important that people understand the probability of a hazard such as the side effect of a treatment occurring but it is also important that it is clear whether a risk is 'relative' or 'absolute'. Figures such as 1 in 1000 or 3 in 100, represent the absolute risk of something occurring, where the absolute risk is the number of new cases of a disease that develop during a specified period divided by the number of disease-free subjects at risk of developing the disease at the beginning of that period (Greener 1996). However, risk may also be referred to as 'relative' and is used when comparing two groups of people, for example the risk of non-smokers developing lung cancer compared to the risk of smokers developing lung cancer. Relative risk may appear to increase substantially but if only a small number of people are affected then the absolute risk remains small (Greener 1996). To illustrate this Gigerenzer and Edwards (2003: 741) use the example of breast screening, showing that if women aged over 50 years of age undergo breast screening they reduce the risk of dying of breast cancer by 25 per cent, however, in terms of absolute risk this actually only represents a risk reduction of 1 in 1000, because of 1000 women aged over 50 who are not screened about 4 will die from breast cancer within 10 years, whereas in a screened population of 1000 women 3 will die. Relative risk can therefore be misleading and may suggest to the lay person that treatments or interventions are more (or less) successful than they are actually are.

Risk assessment does not take place in a vacuum but in the social, cultural, economic and political world, where people are influenced by a wide array of factors, this model of risk perception, the psychometric model, makes the assumption that risk is subjectively defined by individuals (Casiday 2007). Associated with risk perception is a language of risk which includes words such as avoidable, justifiable, acceptable and seriousness (Calman 1996). A risk may be avoidable or unavoidable and where it is avoidable there is a degree of choice as an individual, group or organisation may choose whether or not to accept a risk or change or modify their behaviour to avoid that risk. In some circumstances a risk may be considered to be justifiable but not in others, similarly a risk may be thought to be acceptable or unacceptable except in extreme circumstances, and a risk may be perceived as serious or non-serious. Some risks are deemed more 'acceptable' than others and will be undertaken in the anticipation that some benefit may be gained; this may help to explain why people will often accept much higher risks if the activity involved is voluntary and something they want to do. For example, in 'extreme' sports such as BASE jumping, jet skiing and snowboarding, it is often the fact that they are dangerous and carry a high risk that makes them exciting and therefore appealing. Slovic (1987) reported that individuals will accept risks one thousand times greater from voluntary activities than from hazards which are imposed upon them. Those who ignore known health risks are not only placing themselves in danger of illness and disability but may expose others to harm and place a burden on health and social services. Increasingly, heavy smokers and heavy drinkers and the overweight are stigmatised by society, because of their high risk behaviours which are seen to contribute to patterns of ill health (Wainwright 2008). There have been debates in the media as to whether obese people, alcoholics and smokers should have the same right of access to services as other people on the basis that they have brought the condition on themselves through irresponsible lifestyle choices. The issues surrounding the rights of individuals to treatment is explored in depth by Ellis in Chapter 1 and the question of where responsibility lies for maintaining good health is examined further below.

Increasing pressure on health and social care resources due to the increasing population and fiscal restraints due to economic difficulties creates an ethical and moral dilemma – should treatment and access to services be rationed on the basis of how 'deserving' or 'undeserving' a person is perceived to be?

In considering your position on this ask yourself the following questions:

■ Is it the responsibility of the individual to avoid known health risks for their self-preservation?

■ What measures should be taken against 'high risk takers' to limit the impact of their actions on the rest of society?

■ How much control should the state have in controlling people's life choices – is it the responsibility of the state to undertake this role?

The responses to such questions will produce a range of opinions and perspectives. At one end of the spectrum there is a libertarian perspective which would describe any attempt by governments to control individual behaviours as paternalistic, and interfering with the individuals' right to makes choices about lifestyle regardless of the impact on the wider community. At the other end is the view that everyone has the duty or an obligation to society to keep themselves as healthy as possible, and should take all reasonable measures to achieve this. Although such perspectives are in opposition to each other both may result in the individual being blamed for their own ill health and as therefore being considered as 'undeserving'.

Responsibility for health?

Although access to health care is not necessarily a 'right', according to the World Health Organisation (1978), health itself is a fundamental human right. As life expectancy has increased so has the value attributed to good health, and there is some expectation in modern society that people will take responsibility for their own health and will remain fit for work as ill health resulting in unemployment is placing pressure on society and resources. Risks to health and well-being can be considered as coming from two sources; first, there are external risks from sources such as environmental hazards, over which the individual has little control; secondly, there are internal hazards which are due to individual behaviours and life choices, where the individual is able to exercise some control (Lupton 1995) and also take some responsibility for their actions. Both external and internal factors may influence quality of life, and living a long and healthy life may be considered as a shared responsibility of the individual and the state.

There is an expectation that the government has a responsibility to manage the external risk factors and will protect our environment and inform us, and take action against any risks that emerge, for example by maintaining safe water supplies, and maintaining roads to reduce the risk of road traffic accidents.

As individuals we are encouraged to be risk aware and to make healthy choices to protect our health, to eat a healthy diet, exercise regularly, to avoid smoking and drinking too much alcohol, be vaccinated and attend for screening when invited. We have the right to make our own decisions regarding health behaviours and lifestyle choices but associated with this right is also the responsibility for the wider community. Failing to be vaccinated increases the risks to others of contracting a disease, becoming obese potentially leads to increased costs to the NHS through the need for specialised equipment and possible surgery. We are invited to attend for screening for a number of life-threatening conditions, and to be vaccinated against the potentially serious diseases. Such encouragement is given and promoted through the use of posters and leaflets displayed in public places and in the media. Successive governments have launched health promotion strategies, such as health advice and information, health screening, and vaccinations in the hope not only of increasing life expectancy and reducing morbidity in the population but also in recognition that treating some diseases and conditions is both costly for the NHS and the individual and in some cases of limited efficacy.

Screening actively seeks to identify a disease or pre-disease condition in people who are thought to be and consider themselves to be healthy (Holland and Stewart 1990: 1–2). There are a range of programmes in place in the United Kingdom (see http://www.cancerscreening.nhs.uk) which offer screening for bowel, breast and cervical cancer. Furthermore, there is also screening for conditions besides cancer; for example, prenatal screening for foetal anomalies, sickle cell disease and thalassaemia, abdominal aortic aneurysm (see http://www.screening.nhs.uk). In 2009 a further national programme, NHS Health Checks was introduced to 'predict and prevent' heart disease, stroke, diabetes and kidney disease, in people aged between 40 and 74 years of age (http://www.healthcheck.nhs.uk/), with a five-yearly recall. The rationale behind the scheme it that by identifying risk of these conditions early measures can be taken to reduce the risk and improve the chance of maintaining or improving health in later life.

Screening for cancer is based on the premise that by diagnosing disease at an early stage before symptoms appear the risk of early death is reduced (Baggott 2000). With screening there is, however, also the potential for harm, pathology may be missed (false negative), this may lead to a poorer prognosis and result in litigation. There is a risk of 'over diagnosis' whereby a disease is detected which would not normally become apparent during the person's lifetime; this could have a psychological impact on the person who thought they were healthy, it may also lead to unnecessary treatment and surgery with the associated risks. Another risk is that of false positives leading to anxiety and further diagnostic tests including biopsies which could lead to side effects and complications. When people are screened 'incidentalomas' may be observed; these are findings of uncertain significance, but generally require further investigation which has implications not only for the patient but also for the NHS in terms of additional resource use (Berrington de Gonzalez 2007). Faith or belief in test results may lead to a false sense of security, and if symptoms do appear, they may be ignored because the scan was 'normal'. Moreover, if a person is told they are 'healthy' they may continue with poor lifestyle choices and also may not go to the doctor if symptoms do develop on the basis of being given the all clear. In addition to these risks, breast screening uses ionising radiation (x-rays) and therefore has a further hazard associated with it. The current estimated risks from diagnostic x-rays have been calculated from research on the survivors of the atomic bombings of Hiroshima and Nagasaki at the end of the Second World War, and the nuclear plant accident at Chernobyl in the 1980s. That being said the UK National Health Service Breast Screening Programme (NHSBSP) reviewed the risks and benefits of using ionising radiation to screen for breast cancer, estimating the numbers of cancers detected by screening and the numbers of lives saved, and also the number of lives lost due to radiation induced cancers. It calculated that the ratio of lives saved to lost is approximately 100:1; that is, the benefit of screening exceeds the risk of a radiation induced cancer one hundred times, and that the risk of a radiation-induced cancer for a woman attending mammographic screening by the NHSBSP is about 1 in 20,000 per visit (NHSBSP 2003). Therefore the benefit of undergoing breast screening appears to outweigh the risk due to exposure to radiation, and women are encouraged to be 'breast aware' and to attend regularly for breast screening to take care of their own well-being. In the leaflet that women receive with their invitation for breast screening (NHSBSP 2010) the advantages of breast screening are listed as to prevent death from breast cancer, to find breast cancer early, and to reduce likelihood of mastectomy and chemotherapy. Despite this the take-up rate for breast screening is not 100 per cent, indeed in 2008–2009 the uptake of breast screening was 73.7 per cent, with more than a quarter of eligible women not attending for breast screening (NHSBSP 2010).

There are a number of reasons why people may choose not to be screened, they may believe that they personally are not at risk or they may prefer not to know. In conditions such as breast cancer there is always a degree of uncertainty associated with the likelihood of developing the disease. There is currently a 1 in 8 risk of women living in the UK developing breast cancer in their lifetime (CancerHelp 2011), but although there are certain risk factors attributed to an increased risk, for example age and family history, the uncertainty surrounding as to which individual will be the 'one in eight' enables some people to rationalise the risk. They may argue that it 'won't happen to them', as they have no family history and therefore have 'good genes', they have a sensible diet, don't drink much alcohol, don't smoke, and they have never taken oral contraceptives. If people can counter the known risk factor with such arguments, they may not consider themselves to be at risk of a disease. Others have a 'fatalistic approach' which is one of resigned acceptance that events should be allowed to take their course (Giddens 1991: 112) and see their health as something that they can have no control over and that no matter what they do they may still succumb to an illness.

> People often have a fatalistic attitude towards risk because they have observed that life does not always 'play by the rules'. Someone who drinks heavily and smokes may live to a ripe old age, whilst an ascetic non-smoking, jogging, vegetarian may die young. (Lupton 1999: 111)

━━━━━━━━━━━━━━━━━━━━ **CHALLENGE** ━━━━━━━━━━━━━━━━━━━━

Can you think of a time when you have weighed up your risk of contracting or developing a disease, or the risks associated with continuing with a lifestyle choice (such as smoking, alcohol consumption, 'safe sex')?

▪ What is your own attitude to risk has it changed over time?

▪ How does it affect your decision making in relation to health and lifestyle?

Now consider a person that you have looked after or had responsibility for – did their attitude to risk have an influence on the care or advice that you gave to them?

━━

Although some people choose not to be screened, others 'the worried well' seek out other additional forms and sources of medical screening. Some private medical companies offer health assessments including Computerised Tomography (CT) screening. In the early 2000s there was a trend for some centres to offer whole-body screening, and in 2007 Saga Insurance were offering their customers the opportunity to undergo Saga health screening including a 'Saga Multiscan' which included CT of the heart and colon (Wald 2007). In 2009 Tesco were offering their customers the opportunity to use their clubcard reward points to purchase a health check; on the website it was advertised as a personal 'MOT' describing it as

> The straightforward process uses advanced open CT scanning technology to take high resolution images of your vital organs. The images are so detailed they can reveal the early signs of heart disease, lung cancer, colon cancer, aneurysms, osteoporosis and other illnesses. Catch them early, and they can be treated quickly and effectively. (Reproduced on the Society of Radiographers website 2009)

When this screening first became available and was advertised in the media the providers of these services emphasised the benefits of early diagnosis but no mention was made of the associated risks of CT scans. The Department of Health launched an inquiry to assess whether the so-called health MOTs using body scans offered benefits that outweigh the risks caused by exposure to radiation. The resultant report by the Committee on Medical Aspects of Radiation in the Environment (COMARE 2007) made a number of recommendations including: whole body scanning of asymptomatic patients should stop as there is insufficient evidence to justify the exposure; CT scanning should only take place of anatomical regions where there is evidence of its diagnostic value; and information should be provided by the commercial services regarding the dose and risk of the initial CT scan. As a result of this the providers have modified the information they provide outlining the radiation risks and they also apply inclusion and exclusion criteria to the procedures to limit access.

It could be argued that allowing people to purchase this screening is a matter of personal liberty, as it could be reassuring and enables them to take control of their health. However, to make an informed choice it is necessary to understand the potential risks associated with such procedures, especially if the opportunity is being offered by trusted institutions such as an insurance company and a supermarket chain. There is also an economic and ethical dimension in that if people can afford to choose this service then they should be allowed to, but who should then pay for any additional tests or procedures that are required as a result of the screening and who should be responsible for organising them? If the person does not have medical insurance should they then get the necessary treatment on the NHS ahead of people who are symptomatic and have been waiting for diagnostic tests in NHS hospitals?

The majority of eligible adults are able to make informed choices as to whether or not to attend for screening and in all screening programmes there are a significant number of non-attenders. There are, however, instances where the decision whether to attend is not straightforward – for example, people who have severe physical disabilities and those with learning disabilities. All people regardless of their disabilities have the same rights to access to health promotion services as the rest of the population, for those with physical disabilities transport and access to facilities may be difficult and they may be reliant on others to support them in their actions. For those with learning disabilities it is important that they are able to understand what the screening process entails to enable them to make a decision whether or not they wish to attend. The following case study highlights some of the issues surrounding rights for those with learning disabilities and their access to health care.

CASE STUDY

Sara Mead is a 21-year-old woman with profound learning disabilities. She is able communicate at a very simple level and her understanding of the world around her appears to be very limited. Although she lives in residential care, she has regular contact with her family and her mother visits her 2 or 3 times a week. As Sara has recently had her 21st birthday she is now eligible for cervical cancer screening and the carers in the home believe that as life for people with profound disabilities should be as normal as possible Sara should enter the screening programme and the care home manager makes an appointment for Sara to attend. In recognition of the rights of disabled people to have the same access to screening as others, (where access is both the physical access of the venue and facilities and also access to information to enable them to make their own decisions as to whether or not to accept the invitation for

➡

➜

screening), the NHS Screening Service published guidance for health care professionals working in the service, *Equal access to breast and cervical screening for disabled women* (NHSBSP/CSP 2006). To support this guidance, resources in the form of picture books have been designed for women with learning disabilities to inform them about the screening programmes, further picture books are available to help to decide whether to attend, to help prepare for it, and to understand results and what further investigations may be done. When Sara's mother, Mrs Mead, sees the booklets in her daughter's care notes, and realises that the appointment has been made she is horrified as she believes that her daughter would find the experience extremely distressing and traumatic, and believes that as her daughter is not known to be sexually active that the risk to Sara in terms of the stress and the potential for physical trauma if she struggled during the procedure would outweigh any likelihood of discovering cervical cancer. She complains to the manager and raises her concerns. However, because Sara is over the age of 18 and is therefore an adult her mother cannot refuse or cancel the examination on Sara's behalf, and the home care manager does not change the appointment for the smear test despite her mother's objections.

Under the Mental Capacity Act (2005) every adult should be assumed to have capacity to make a particular decision unless it is established that they lack capacity to do so. To support and encourage decision making it states that every effort should be made to present information in a relevant way so that it is easier for the individual to understand (see Koubel and Yardley, Chapter 4, for a more in-depth analysis of the Mental Capacity Act). Although the carers in the home believe Sara does understand the implications of having the test Mrs Mead is not convinced that her daughter fully understands what the smear test involves, and is concerned that if the test goes ahead and Sara was restrained in some way during the process it would infringe her civil liberties and could constitute abuse. She therefore complains to the Local Authority who run the home, demanding that the appointment is cancelled. According to the Code of Practice (Department of Constitutional Affairs 2007) developed to accompany the Mental Capacity Act 2005, where there is a disagreement between professionals and a person's family regarding their personal welfare then it is recommended that an informal discussion with all those involved should take place and that independent expert advice should be taken to consider the best interests of the person involved. A case conference was therefore convened involving Sara, her mother and all those health and social care professionals involved in her care.

One of the key principles of the Mental Capacity Act is that any act done to or any decision made on behalf of a person who lacks capacity must be done or made in that person's best interests, but working out what is in someone else's best interests can be difficult. At the conference the care home manager argues that Sara should have the opportunity to be screened on both Kantian and utilitarian ethical grounds. First, she stresses the moral obligation to screen all eligible women regardless of their disability because cervical cancer screening is an effective way of identifying early stage cervical cancer and thus can reduce the impact of treatment and improve prognosis. The

➜

➜

manager also is concerned that people with profound learning disabilities should have the same rights to health care as the rest of the population and there is therefore a duty to screen Sara, and to enable her to be included in the normal processes of everyday living. This 'normalising' of a person may appear laudable but it may also be considered as using Sara as a means of achieving the manager's aims rather than considering her individual and specific needs. On the other hand, Mrs Mead has based her opinion on her judgement as to the probable outcomes of attempting the test (an act utilitarian perspective – Beauchamp and Childress 1994: 51). From Mrs Mead's perspective it is unlikely that Sara would comply with requirements of the procedure; it would be distressing for her, and the probability of discovering a cancer would be low, and as such it would not be in Sara's best interests to be screened. The Code of Practice specifies that the final decision for what is in the best interests of the person lacking in capacity is the member of the health care team responsible for the person's treatment, the decision-maker. In this case the General Practitioner (GP) would be the person responsible for the smear test and if the GP considers that if the probability is that the test will be successfully accomplished and that a possible diagnosis is the discovery of a cancer, with risks of undertaking the procedure minimal, then there is an obligation to treat Sara in the same way as other 21-year-olds. However, the GP knows that the incidence of cervical cancer has been falling since the 1980s, that it accounts for only 2 per cent of all female cancers, and that those most of risk of developing the disease are sexually active and smokers (Cancer Research UK 2003) and that therefore Sara would be at low risk of developing the disease. The GP has also had to treat Sara on other occasions and knows that during visits to the surgery she has become visibly distressed and agitated. Having listened to both Mrs Mead and the manager's arguments he asks Sara to look at the leaflets about the test and asks her questions to try and gain an understanding of her awareness as to what is involved. As a result of these discussions the GP concludes that Sara is not sufficiently aware of what she would experience and that it would not be in her best interests for her to be screened.

CHALLENGE

■ Do you agree with this decision?

■ If not why do you think Sara should be screened?

If the manager and carers disagreed with this decision they could apply to the Court of Protection (http://www.publicguardian.gov.uk/index.htm); you may find this website useful for more information about the Code of Practice and the legal position regarding capacity and making decisions for other people.

With all diagnostic investigations including screening there is a balance between the risk and benefits of undergoing such tests. Whilst the majority of people support the concept of screening for cancer and other conditions before they become 'too serious', prenatal screening for genetic abnormalities and foetal anomalies does raise ethical and moral questions and the issue of rights. Prenatal or antenatal screening has become part of routine care in the UK and there is an expectation that pregnant women will attend antenatal appointments where their own health and the growth and development of the foetus are monitored. A woman who fails to attend appointments may be blamed if the child is born with a disability, as she is considered to have responsibility for looking after herself during pregnancy for the sake of her family, society and the unborn child (Beck-Gernsheim 2000).

CHALLENGE

Consider the following two statements (adapted from Gillott 2001) and think about the arguments for and against each position:

■ Antenatal screening and testing is wrong because it devalues those living with a disability.

■ Antenatal screening and testing is a biological approach to a biological problem. People who choose to terminate a pregnancy because of foetal abnormalities are not making a moral judgement about those living with a disability.

Prenatal screening may lead to selective abortion in response to the diagnosis of a foetal abnormality; such decisions may be based on a number of factors including on the basis of best interests of the child and the mother, and judgements may be made regarding the individual's potential quality of life. However, there is also concern that such screening is also undertaken to produce so-called 'designer babies' and may be considered eugenic. It is suggested by some disability rights advocates that prenatal diagnosis of a disability which may lead to termination of the pregnancy is a form of discrimination against the disabled (Gillam 1999), because from the perspective of the Disability Rights Movement, living with a disability need not be detrimental to the possibility of living a worthwhile and valued existence.

It is not only screening which raises issues about risks, rights and responsibilities in health promotion. The vaccination programme has also produced controversies around rights and personal liberty since the introduction of the first vaccines in the early 1800s (Wolfe and Sharpe, 2002). Compulsory vaccination for smallpox in the nineteenth century led to anti-vaccination protests by those who saw it as an infringement of civil liberties and as stigmatising the poor (Hobson-West 2007). Compulsory vaccination conflicts with individual rights to make choices as to how to maintain health; currently in the UK there are no compulsory vaccinations, unlike the USA and France where children cannot start state primary schools without vaccination certificates (Clements and Ratzan 2003). In the UK vaccinations are delivered free of charge by the NHS according to a prescribed immunisation schedule ('The Green Book', Salisbury *et al.* 2006), and parents are strongly encouraged to have their children vaccinated through the use of promotional literature such as leaflets, posters, information packs, factsheets and websites.

The primary aim of any vaccination is to protect the person who receives the vaccination, it also means that vaccinated people are less likely to be a source of infection to others and thus reduce the risk of others who are unvaccinated being exposed to that infection. This is known as herd or population immunity and operates because the proportion of people susceptible to infection in a group that are in physical contact is so low that transmission is unlikely. It means that those people who cannot be vaccinated also benefit from vaccination programmes; however, for herd immunity to be effective there needs to be a certain number of people within the population who are vaccinated (Rogers and Pilgrim 1995). Health care professionals have a vested interested in ensuring vaccinations are carried out as the GP practice is rewarded for achieving 70 per cent and 90 per cent coverage of their practice population.

When making decisions as to whether or not to have their child vaccinated, parents have the right to be informed about the risks and benefits. Information regarding the risks associated with undertaking (or not) the various health promoting procedures and treatments is evidence based, but how this information is communicated is problematical (Alaszewski 2005). First, risk assessments by professionals are generally based on population studies and not on the individual concerned, whereas for a parent deciding as to whether or not to have their child vaccinated their concern may be around the risk of their particular child having an adverse reaction to the vaccination, rather than the risk of the child contracting the disease, or protecting others in the community through herd immunity. This may be in part due to the falling incidence of common childhood diseases leading to a lack of awareness of the potential serious consequences of these diseases. Risk assessments are also based on past events and there is therefore a degree of uncertainty as to the extent to which future events can be predicated on the past. Secondly, communication is increasingly a two-way process with more people adopting an active role, for example 'the expert patient', and using external sources such as the internet, and the experiences of families and friends to inform their decisions. People are also less trusting of experts and 'expert knowledge' following recent scandals in the NHS such as the children's heart surgery inquiry (Bristol Inquiry 2000, Kennedy 2001) the Royal Liverpool Children's Inquiry (Alder Hey Report, Redfern *et al.* 2001) and the Harold Shipman case in 2005. The fact that people know that doctors are paid to reach targets for vaccination also has implications for the trust relationship between parents and the GPs.

Lack of consensus between so-called experts also reduces the public's trust in the efficacy and effectiveness of medicine. The debates in the medical press and the media triggered by the *Lancet* article by Dr Andrew Wakefield (Wakefield *et al.* 1998) raised concern over the safety of the MMR (Mumps Measles Rubella) vaccine. Wakefield's research linked the MMR vaccine with an increased risk of autism and inflammatory bowel disease; however, the research was based on a very small sample size and its findings were contested by the medical community. The media coverage surrounding the controversy was high and in subsequent years the numbers of children vaccinated fell (and the number of MMR cases reported rose). In a large study looking at immunisation the reasons parents gave for not having their children immunised included concerns about safety, risks of vaccine outweighing the risks of contracting the disease, negative publicity, and not trusting the advice given by health care professionals or the government (Pearce *et al.* 2008). Therefore to increase levels of vaccination in the population health care providers will need to overcome such parental concerns. However, there are a number of potential difficulties with this, including the fact that as the number of people who are immunised against a disease increases the fewer cases of the disease will occur and the risk of serious symptoms and complications of the illness will also become smaller, but the risks associated with being vaccinated will increase on an individual level (Rogers and Pilgrim 1995), so the perceived risks of vaccination may appear greater than contracting the disease. Some diseases, such as small pox, have been eradicated through vaccination and this would be the overall goal of any vaccination programme, but this would be difficult to achieve without compulsory vaccinations, which again raises issues around personal rights and liberties.

CHALLENGE

■ Do you think vaccinations should be compulsory in the UK?

■ How could people be persuaded to be vaccinated or have their child vaccinated?

■ If people refuse vaccination what sanctions do you think (if any) should be put in place? (Stop child benefit? Refuse entry to school?)

Conclusion

This chapter has looked at the statistical measures of risk and considered the scientific approach to risk, and the different ways in which risk is defined. There then follows an exploration of the rights and responsibilities around the different strategies for maintaining health and preventing disease. In conclusion, promoting health and well-being has risks, rights and responsibilities associated with it. Whilst we can argue that the government has a responsibility to protect its citizens' health and well-being through environmental measures and the provision of health and social care services, as individuals we have the right to access health care services and a responsibility to ourselves and society to maintain our own health through having a healthy lifestyle and attending the health promotion services and opportunities available to us. In the following chapter there is an in-depth exploration of the shifting nature of responsibility for health between the state and the individual over the past century, clarifying the reasons why responsibility for maintaining health is currently very much with the individual.

References

Alaszewski, A. (2005) A person-centred approach to communicating risk. *PLoS Medicine* 2(2): 41.

Baggott, R. (2000) *Public Health: Policy and Politics*. Basingstoke: Macmillan Press.

Beck, U. (1999) *World Risk Society*. Cambridge: Polity Press.

Beck-Gernsheim, E. (2000) Health and responsibility: from social change to technological change and vice versa. In B. Adam, U. Beck, J. Van Loon (eds), *The Risk Society and Beyond*. London: Sage.

Beauchamp, T. L. and Childress, J. F. (1994) *Principles of Biomedical Ethics* (4th edn). Oxford: Oxford University Press

Berrington de Gonzalez, A. (2007) Computed Tomography screening: safe and effective? *Journal of Medical Screening*, 14(4): 165–67.

Calman, K. C. (1996) Cancer: science and society and the communication of risk. *British Medical Journal*, 313: 799–802.

Calman, K. C. and Royston, G. (1997) Risk language and dialects. *British Medical Journal*, 315: 939 (cited in Department of Health 1997).

CancerHelp UK (2011) Breast cancer risks and causes. Available at: http://www. cancerhelp.org.uk/type/breast-cancer/about/risks/ (accessed 22 January 2011).

Casiday, R. E. (2007) Children's health and social theory of risk: insights from the British measles, mumps and rubella (MMR) controversy. *Social Science & Medicine*, 65: 1059–70.

Cancer Research UK (2003) *Cervical Cancer UK*. Available at: http://publications.cancerresearchuk.org/WebRoot/crukstoredb/CRUK_PDFs/ CSCERV03.pdf

Clements, C. J. and Ratzan, S. (2003) Misled and confused? Telling the public about MMR vaccine safety. *Journal of Medical Ethics*, 29: 22–6.

Committee on Medical Aspects of Radiation in the Environment (COMARE) (2007) Twelfth Report, *The Impact of Personally Initiated X-ray Computed Tomography Scanning for the Health Assessment of Asymptomatic Individuals*, Health Protection Agency. Available at: http://www.comare.org.uk/comare_docs.htm#statements

Department of Health (1997) *Communicating about Risks to Public Health: Pointers to Good Practice*. Available at: http://www.dh.gov.uk/en/Publicationsandstatistics/ Publications/PublicationsPolicyAndGuidance/DH_4006604 (accessed 21 November 2010).

Douglas, M. (1992) *Risk and Blame: Essays in Cultural Theory*. London: Routledge.

European Commission (1998) *A Guideline on the Readability of the Label and Package Leaflet of Medicinal Products for Human Use*. EC Pharmaceuticals Committee.

Giddens, A. (1991) *Modernity and self-identity*. Cambridge: Polity Press.

Gigerenzer, G. and Edwards, A. (2003) Simple tools for understanding risk: from innumeracy to insight. *British Medical Journal*, 327: 741–4.

Gillam, L. (1999) Prenatal diagnosis and discrimination against the disabled. *Journal of Medical Ethics*, 25: 163–71.

Gillott, J. (2001) Screening for disability: a eugenic pursuit? *Journal of Medical Ethics*, 27 (supplement): 21–3.

Greener, D. (1996) Putting risk in perspective. *Practice Nursing*, 7(20): 13–16.

Hobson-West, P. (2007) 'Trusting blindly can be the biggest risk of all': organised resistance to childhood vaccination in the UK. *Sociology of Health and Illness*, 29(2): 198–215.

Holland, W. W. and Stewart, S. (1990) *Screening in Health Care: Benefit or Bane?* London: The Nuffield Provincial Hospitals Trust.

Knapp, P., Raynor, D. K. and Berry, D. C. (2004) Comparison of two methods of presenting risk information to patients about the side effects of medicines. *Quality and Safety in Health Care* 13: 176–80.

Lupton, D. (1995) *The Imperative of Health: Public Health and the Regulated Body*. London: Sage.

Lupton, D. (1999) *Risk*. London: Routledge.

Mythen, G. (2004) *Ulrich Beck: A Critical Introduction to the Risk Society*. London: Pluto Press.

NHSBSP (2003) *Review of Risk Radiation in Breast Screening*, Report by a joint working party of the NHSBSP National Coordinating Group for Physics Quality Assurance and the National Radiological Protection Board, NHSBSP Publication No 54.

NHSBSP/CSP (2006) *Equal Access to Breast and Cervical Screening for Disabled Women*. NHS Cancer Screening Programme. Available at: http://www.cancerscreening.nhs.uk/publications/cs2.pdf (accessed 14 January 2011).

NHSBSP (2010) *Annual Review*. Available at: http://www.cancerscreening.nhs.uk/breastscreen/publications/nhsbsp-annualreview2010.pdf

Office of National Statistics (2008) www.ons.gov.uk

Paling, J. (2003) Strategies to help patients understand risks. *British Medical Journal*, 327: 745–8.

Pearce, A., Law, C., Elliman, D., Cole, T. and Bedford, H. (2008) Factors associated with uptake of measles, mumps, and rubella vaccine (MMR) and use of single antigen vaccines in a contemporary UK cohort: prospective cohort study. *British Medical Journal*, 336(7747): 754–60.

Redfern, M., Keeling, J. W. and Powell, E. (2001) *The Royal Liverpool Children's Inquiry (Alder Hey Report)*. London: The Stationery Office. Available at: http://www.rlcinquiry.org.uk

Rogers, A. and Pilgrim, D. (1995) The risk of resistance: perspectives on the mass childhood immunisation programme. In J. Gabe (ed.), *Medicine Health and Risk*. Oxford: Blackwell.

Salisbury, D., Ramsay, M. and Noakes, K. (2006) *Immunisation against Infectious Disease: 'The Green Book'*. Norwich: The Stationery Office. Available at: www.dh.gov.uk/en/Policyandguidance/Healthandsocialcaretopics/Greenbook/DH_4097254.

Society of Radiographers (2009) Society takes on Tesco, 21 May. Available at: http://www.sor.org/stories/society-takes-tesco (accessed 18 December 2010).

Slovic, P. (1987) Perception of risk. *Science*, 236: 280–5.

Wainwright, D. (ed.) (2008) *A Sociology of Health*. London: Sage.

Wakefield, A., Murch, S., Anthony, A., Linnell, J., Casson, D., Malik, M., Berelowitz, M., Dhillon, A. P., Thomson, M. A., Harvey, P., Valentine, A., Davies, S. E. and Walker-Smith, J. A. (1998) Ileal-lymphoid-nodular hyperplasia, non-specific colitis, and pervasive developmental disorder in children. *Lancet*, 351(9103): 637–41.

Wald, N. J. (2007) Screening – a step too far: a matter of concern. *Journal of Medical Screening*, 14(4): 163–4.

Wolfe, R. M. and Sharp, L. K. (2002) Anti-vaccinationists past and present. *British Medical Journal*, 325: 430–2.

World Health Organisation (1946) *Constitution: Basic Documents*. Geneva: World Health Organisation.

World Health Organisation (1978) *Declaration of Alma Ata: Report of the International Conference on Primary Health Care*. Geneva: WHO/Unicef.

Rights, Risks and Responsibilities in an Age of Uncertainty

Adrian Adams

Introduction

Over the last 20 years an awareness of the presence of risk has come to dominate and shape our experience of both our natural and social environments. This sense that we now live in a 'risk society' (Beck 1992), is closely associated with a lack of confidence in the capacity of governments and institutions to protect our public and private lives from the apparently unpredictable and unavoidable impact of an increasing range and severity of unforeseen hazards in a globalised world, for example from the effects of global warming, economic failures and terrorist attacks.

More immediately, in Western democratic societies that have become accustomed to the security provided by the provisions of a welfare state, the shifting balance between the role of the state and the responsibility of individuals, has significantly impacted upon services and practices in health and social care institutions and organisations. This in turn has increased our sensitivity to the presence of risks and generated a level of anxiety amongst the public and, as commentators such as Frank Furedi (2008) have claimed, particularly amongst parents, to such an extent that we now appear to be more preoccupied with the risks that surround and penetrate our lives, than with the routine activities of family and social life, from which we draw meaning, purpose and pleasure (Luhmann 1996).

As it becomes apparent that the welfare state as it was originally envisaged is not sustainable, so our pre-occupation with risk management and cost effectiveness in a system driven by market principles has profound implications for the nature of collective welfare in general, and for the purpose and ethical basis of health and social care services. Current trends within the welfare system exemplify how:

> in the West, our moral codes have become focused more on a concern for control than for care, for regulating one another rather than caring for one another. (Burkitt 1997: 151)

Whilst in the previous chapter Bungay explored risk assessment using mainly a scientific approach, this chapter examines how our awareness and understanding of risk intersects with changing attitudes towards rights and responsibilities and how these have changed over time, reflecting the increased liberalisation of society in the United Kingdom. In particular, it considers how attempts by successive governments to 'roll back the state' and dismantle the institutions and commitments of the welfare state in favour of a mixed and now market economy of care have shaped public attitudes and expectations.

The chapter also examines how the response from those working in health and social care services to the shift in the nature of the relationship between the state and the individual is largely determined by their role and function as an instrument of government policy.

As the debate over how we should approach matters of risk, rights and responsibility has increasingly been reduced to the technical and bureaucratic level, so too have broader ideological and moral considerations been stripped out of debates over what welfare means in and for society. It is therefore argued here that health and social care professionals should understand that the notions of risks, rights and responsibilities are ideological constructs and as such should not be taken as 'givens' but should be appreciated as being both contested and subject to social and political influences.

The chapter concludes with reference to the need for a renewed and refreshed approach to the matter of and relationship between risk, rights and responsibilities in health and social care at a time of heightened insecurity and uncertainty. It claims that there is now a pressing need to develop processes for increasing trust and reflection across society and for more sophisticated approaches to professional interventions in complex policy areas and practice situations.

LEARNING OUTCOMES

By the end of the chapter you should have developed your understanding of:

- How our sense of self is developed through our relationships with others

- The notions of citizenship and the responsibility that comes with being a citizen

→

→

- How the state took responsibility for its citizens through the development of the national health and welfare services during the twentieth century

- The shift back to individual responsibility and risk management in the late twentieth and early twenty-first centuries

- How health and social care practitioners' responses to rights, risks and responsibilities have been shaped by political ideologies.

Fundamental considerations in the relationship between individuals and society

To help us understand the relationship between the state and the individual, we should first consider the notion of personhood (Koubel and Bungay 2009). There is considerable diversity across human societies and cultures regarding the nature of personhood, in child rearing, socialisation and in types of social relationships. However, underlying this variety of beliefs and behaviours regarding how we develop as a person and take up our place in society there is a shared sense that who we are – that is, our identity – is formed and develops through the relationships we establish with other people. It is in this way we come to know who we are from whom we are connected to and with whom we share a sense of belonging, as members of a family, group or community. However, our sense of self is also shaped by reference to those who we perceive as being different from us and who represent not only a difference, but also a potential threat in as much as they do not necessarily share our sentiments, beliefs or commitments.

The relationships we have with others, as being ones of either sameness or difference, are both cognitive in that they have been taught and learnt, and affective in that they are emotional and felt; so that we simultaneously both know and experience who we are like and who we are different from. Our relationships thus shape our behaviour towards and our expectations of other people. Within the social environment these expectations and behaviours are captured and reflected through a variety of forms of social exchanges and moral practices expressed as entitlements and obligations, rights and responsibilities, that become formalised through cultural, political, legal, bureaucratic and professional codes, processes and procedures. Risks are considered to arise when individuals fall out of this web of social exchanges in that they do not receive the exchange of duties and benefits of being a member of 'society' because for some reason they do not meet the prevailing socio-cultural expectations regarding what they are entitled to or responsible for.

Can you identify a person who you think has had the most influence on you in your:

■ personal or family life

■ education

■ working life.

How has this person had an impact on your behaviour, attitudes, expectations or aspirations?

Why was this person able to influence you?

Each of the social sciences offers us a particular view of how human identity is constructed through the relationship between the individual and the group, a relationship that shapes our understanding of and emotional response to others as being like or unlike ourselves. Sociological, anthropological and psychological theory all refer back in their own unique ways to this basic assumptions about human identity. For example, Mary Douglas (1970), an anthropologist, introduced the two interrelated concepts of 'group' and 'grid' as determining how firstly an individual's social position is determined as being either inside or outside a particular social group and secondly how an individual's social role is defined through networks of social privileges, claims and obligations. The social psychologists Michael Hogg and Dominic Abrams (1998), building on the research of Henri Tajfel (1981) argue for a social identity approach to explain the operations of intergroup relations, prejudice and discrimination and the impact of groups on individual identity. Norbet Elias, the German sociologist, argued that individual psychic structures are moulded by social attitudes, or as he puts it:

> Society's order, its tensions and constraints, and the openings for change it offers all reside within those relationships between individuals, in other words within networks or figurations. What happens within a figuration is closely related to the psychic make-up, the tensions and constraints, and the openings for change that reside within the very individuals who are part of it. (Elias 2000: 41)

List all the social groups/networks that you belong to (e.g. family, work team, sports club, Facebook).

Ask a friend or colleague to do the same.

What do you think the groups you belong to tell others about you?

The emergence of civic and human rights and responsibilities

Whilst as human beings we are all enmeshed in a web of social relationships and moral obligations which primarily constitute our immediate family and friends, the extent to which these then take on a collective or universal form, to include communities and membership of other social, religious, ethnic, political or occupational groupings allows for considerable diversity amongst different people.

The idea that an individual had formal or public rights and responsibilities originates from the Greek concept of citizenship. Citizenship is based on the assumption that the relationship between people and the communities in which they lived offered benefits to both the individual citizen and the community through conferred rights and responsibilities. As such it also required criteria of exclusivity in that citizenship could only be claimed and taken up on the grounds of meeting certain criteria, for example political participation, the payment of taxes or heritage.

Under the Romans, the notion of citizenship was expanded to include people from across their empire as a means of securing and legitimizing Roman rule over conquered areas and as such emphasised the legal rather than political status of citizenship. By the Middle Ages though, the legal status of citizenship had been lost and citizenship had become more associated with 'city states' applied mainly for the purpose of distinguishing between the aristocracy, the emergent merchant classes and commoners. By the seventeenth century, the idea of rights based on citizenship was revived through the English Bill of Rights 1689, which later served as a model for the United States of America's Bill of Rights 1789. Most notably during this period, the French Revolution (1789–99) swept away many of the feudal, aristocratic and religious privileges, as traditional social hierarchies gave way to principles of citizenship and inalienable rights.

Universal human rights were first recognised internationally in the twentieth century following the end of the Second World War by the Universal Declaration on Human Rights 1948 and the European Convention on Human Rights 1950. More recently, the Human Rights Act 1998 was passed making the human rights in the European Convention on Human Rights directly enforceable in the UK (Donnelly 2003).

Today all modern political-administrative systems (nation states) seek to balance the tensions that arise in society between order and disorder, rationality and passion. The capacity to govern is achieved by imposing a model of either legal-rational authority over or democratic participation by citizens. Governments seek to establish the boundaries of their authority through demarcating who is included and who is excluded as a member of society or citizen and what is acceptable and unacceptable behaviour between citizens. These boundaries are then maintained through a regime of regulation and socialisation delivered through the institutions of society, most notably the family, the school and the welfare system, that include general provisions for ensuring material security, health and social welfare.

It is in this historical context that health and social services, alongside education housing and social security in the UK can be understood as a part of the political-administrative system and an instrument of government intended to shape the rights we are entitled to and responsibilities we are expected to meet as members of society (Powell and Hewitt 2002).

================= **CHALLENGE** =================

As a citizen in the UK we have the right to access health and social care services. In Chapter 1, Ellis explores the 'right' of the citizen further, using a case study approach. You may like to consider at this point what makes a person a citizen of the UK? Is it that they live here? Pay taxes? Were born here? Their parents were born here?

Your answer will help you when considering the rights of citizenship, and the responsibilities of a state to its citizens.

The emergence of risk as a feature of decision making

Just as contemporary assumptions about rights and responsibilities are rooted in and shaped by the historical context that reflects political struggles over resources and authority between competing social groups, so too is our understanding of risk as an emergent notion subject to prevailing beliefs about our ability to interact with and impact upon the natural world and the nature of social relationships.

Niklas Luhmann identifies that the term 'risk' appeared in the English language only in the seventeenth century. It replaced older notions that thought in terms of either fate or good and bad fortune largely (pre)determined outside of direct human influence or as prudence, a virtue to be cultivated which was associated with the emerging world of commerce and market transactions. Luhmann argues that the notion of risk appeared with the transition from traditional to modern society, necessitated by the increasing complexity of perspectives and information that is a feature of the modern world and that makes our knowledge of the future even more uncertain (Luhmann 1996).

Luhmann constructs risk as a 'modern' ability to manage the problems of individual decision making in increasingly complex situations that are a result *not* of nature, god or destiny, as was assumed in premodern societies, but which *are* the result of decisions (Luhmann 1993). He argues that the problem of risk is not so much a matter of facts – that is, that they are determined by the actual dangers arising in the natural environment that must be faced – but rather by the necessity for continuously questioning the risks involved in any decision, which result partly from an unknown future and partly by means of some person's or organisation's risky behaviour.

═══════════════════════ **CHALLENGE** ═══════════════════════

■ How do you define risk?

■ Do your family or friends define it in the same way?

■ Is it always a negative concept?

■ Can you identify any positive consequences of risk?

Your definition and understanding of risk can be an important factor in your assessment and analysis of risk in practice. This will be explored in more depth in subsequent chapters.

Although the future always contains elements of uncertainty and as such there can be no guarantees of safety, only 'risky retreats to safety' (Luhmann 1993), risk is the potential or probability that a chosen action or the choice of inaction will lead to an undesirable outcome. The notion of risk therefore implies that it is the chosen action or choice of inaction that can influence potential loss of a desired outcome. Whilst almost any human endeavour carries some risk, some are much more risky than others. Decision making that incorporates attempts at risk assessment, management and reduction is characterised by the inclusion and calculation of the probabilities associated with any existing threat or danger, inherent vulnerabilities and subsequent impacts arising from action taken.

> If risk is an aspect of decision making, the concept of risk can be defined as the result of an attribution process. It is a construction of an observer. When future possible damages are seen as being caused by a decision, this decision runs a risk – whether or not the negative outcome in fact occurs and whether or not the decision maker takes such a possibility into account or whether it is attributed to him only after the event (one cannot of course avoid risks by ignoring the problem). (Luhmann 1996: 7)

Changes in our understanding of external factors such as God, fate and politics and our awareness of how these affect our lives leads to changes in the way each society constructs the balance of rights, risks and responsibilities. In the following section there is a discussion as to how the UK government took greater responsibility for its citizens' health and well-being through the development of the national health and welfare services through the twentieth century.

The recognition of risk and the provision of social security

The legitimacy and authority of the state to raise taxes and formulate laws derives from its duty to promote and ensure the security, welfare, regulation and progress of the general population. This relationship between the authority and duty of the state and the rights (or entitlements) and responsibilities (or obligations) of citizens is premised on an assumption that there are shared interests between the state and the everyday practical problems of individuals, families and communities.

Accounts of modern health and social care work first appear towards the end of the nineteenth century, among a number of new disciplines whose sentiments and moralities, interests and motives are associated with the project of the enlightenment and the modern era (Giddens 1990). As Foucault has described them:

> During certain periods there appear agents of liaison. Take the example of philanthropy in the early nineteenth century: people appear who make it their business to involve themselves in other people's lives, health, nutrition, housing; then, out of this confused set of functions there emerge certain personages, institutions, forms of knowledge: public hygiene, inspectors, social workers, psychologists. And we are now seeing a whole proliferation of different categories of social work. (Foucault 1980: 62)

Modern health and social services professions took shape from within what Philp (1979) describes as a new 'social space' within society, between the public and the private, where the economic, political and social systems overlapped. This space provided economic and social benefits for the expanding middle class in the form of membership of professional groups such as health and hygiene, law, education, psychiatry and social work (Perkin 1969). Within the expanding political and administrative system health and social services filled a niche among new forms of social regulation and social reform for the management and improvement of individuals and groups whose circumstances and the problems they presented to society could no longer be accommodated by the Poor Laws (Blakemore 2003).

Following the First World War increased attempts were made to establish the common interests and purposes between the state and its citizens, stimulated by continuing concerns over the selectivity of welfare policy and the experience of the interwar economic boom and recession. A limited range of socio-economic policies and legislation were subsequently developed that could in principle be coordinated and administered on a universal and comprehensive basis.

However, the foundations for a welfare state were only fully established as a result of the shared experiences by all sectors of the population arising from the Second World War. The impact of factors such as civilian bombing, rationing, evacuation, the extension and the extended provision of services led to the creation of a social climate and established social attitudes and expectations of a better and more just society with welfare provision for all. These aspirations found public expression in the Beveridge Report (HMSO 1942), which identified the five 'giants' that plagued society: illness, ignorance, disease, squalor and want. To combat these 'giants' the Beveridge Report proposed the creation of a universal state system of welfare 'from cradle to grave' based on a social insurance scheme (Jacobs 1992) which would ensure that everyone would be entitled to gain access to an acceptable minimum standard of health care, education, housing, employment (or unemployment benefit) and social services.

Following the end of the war and the landslide victory of the Labour party in 1945, and in spite of resistance from such bodies as the British Medical Association, legislation was passed to enact Beveridge's plan during the period of the Labour government from 1945–51. Through a series of major pieces of legislation the foundations were laid for the creation of full employment by the adoption of Keynesian (Keynes 1936) economic policies centred on demand management, which attracted cross party support during the period of postwar reconstruction, unprecedented economic growth and high levels of employment. Within a period of 15 years following the end of the Second World War a national health and welfare state system had been established within England based upon the principles and assumptions of welfare outlined by Beveridge and economic growth and stability proposed by Keynes.

The first 30 years of the welfare state from 1945 until the mid 1970s resulted in the creation of services used and valued by the majority of the population. In the welfare state system an accommodation was achieved between the state and the citizenship through the integration of a set of public services that prevented and managed the risks of unemployment, illness and social distress, and a consensus of the respective rights and responsibilities of individual citizens (Hobsbawm 1994). The presumption that the burden of the fundamental risks of labour – that is, accident, illness, loss of employment and lack of provision for old age – could be met by the welfare state was premised upon the aspiration that a peaceful coexistence between democracy and capitalism could be assured through state intervention.

During this period social work played a modest part in the provision of services consisting of a variety of specialist activities provided by distinct occupational groups such as child care officers, mental welfare officers and hospital almoners. The establishment of generic local authority social services departments, through the Local Authority Social Services Act 1970, provided the organisational framework and rationale for social work within the English welfare state model; however, it was the National Health Services that came to represent the commitment of the state to establishing a risk-reducing investment or insurance intended to protect against potential loss of health or social functionality and integration. So, for example, personal risks could be reduced by measures to either prevent or reduce the impact of illness of personal misfortune, which following assessment or diagnosis, could be addressed through the provision of three levels of service: primary prevention actions that decrease early causes of illness or dysfunction; secondary prevention actions after a person has clearly measured clinical or behavioural signs or symptoms recognised as risk factors; tertiary prevention, which is intended to reduce the negative impact of an already established disease or dysfunction by restoring function and reducing disease-related complications (Gilbert and Dunn 2009). (See Chapter 2 for an exploration of the rights, risks and responsibilities surrounding primary prevention measures such as screening and vaccination.)

The erosion of social security under conditions of increasing uncertainty

The presumption that the burden of the fundamental risks that people could encounter in their working lives – that is, accident, illness, loss of employment and lack of provision for old age – could be met by the welfare state was premised upon the aspiration that a peaceful coexistence between democracy and capitalism could be assured through state intervention. This aspiration would be realised through a series of rational interventions by the state into the economic and social systems that affected people's lives.

First, the full employment of all those who could work would be secured, along with the insertion of collective bargaining on wage scales by parties into the economic system. This would be secured by the compensatory mechanisms of the state and through the application of social welfare legislation to the social system. Together these strategies would establish the status of wage earner as the social norm and would be maintained through the processes of political participation, social ownership and the consumption of mass produced goods (Barr 1987).

However, the economic crisis of the 1970s created a situation whereby these presumptions were exposed as false (Offe 1984). The inability of the state to maintain full employment and even some basic services, for example the provision of electric power supplies during the miners' strike and the three-day week, exposed the government of the time as incapable of containing the contradictions between the liberal values of individual liberty, participation and efficiency and the social democratic values of collective solidarity and economic redistribution that were inherent in the notion of a welfare state. Both the new right in central government and the emergent coalitions of the new left within local government, from their separate ideological positions, came up with new definitions of what constituted the basis of the contract between the state and its citizens. Freedom became choice and participation and free access to health and social services a matter of eligibility rather than entitlement, with the community, rather than the state as the arbiter of public services. In effect these radical re-formulations and repudiations of the core tenets of a welfare state system established the possibility for the replacement of universal and substantive benefits *available as of right* by categorical and selective measures of needs to meet defined categories of problems (Cox 1998).

The retreat of government from a commitment to the welfare state and the subsequent development and introduction of a 'Mixed Economy of Welfare' across the economic, social and political/administrative systems was reconstructed and presented as 'Community Care' (Powell and Hewitt 2002). This process of dismantling of the welfare state model also allowed for a discrediting of its bureaucratic and professional infrastructure, which was blamed as a failed attempt to harmonise democracy and capitalism and as being damaging to both. On the one hand, it was claimed that the redistribution of resources through social security payments led to rising wages and benefits, decreased productivity and individual capital accumulation; and on the other, that interventions of regulation, normalisation and surveillance stifled responsibility and initiative amongst the recipients of welfare.

The result was that the postwar political consensus between the two main political parties, Labour and Conservative, that had both sought to achieve the principal objectives of the welfare state, was broken. The project of a state – that is, the collective system that could assume responsibility for intervention within both the economy and the private sphere – was exposed as a flawed and contradictory policy and gave way in favour of an increasingly liberal, that is, individualist approach to insuring against health and social dangers (Offe 1996). In other words, the aspiration, to achieve a balance between social rights, political rights and civil rights did not survive the demise of the welfare state and the slide into a welfare market. Table 3.1 illustrates how the shift in responsibility is linked to ideology and how responsibility has shifted from the individual to the state and back to the individual during the twentieth and twenty-first centuries.

Here, the 'mixed and then later market economy of welfare' has become common shorthand to describe a mixture of state, private, voluntary and informal provision of care for vulnerable individuals, whereby the role and function of state institutions becomes one of enabling rather than providing for the needs of the population as a whole. These changes constituted a radical reformulation of the relationship between the state, the family and the individual, whereby the burden of ensuring social security is shifting away from the state and towards the individual citizen. This shift of responsibility emanates from a belief that the cost of health and social welfare has become prohibitive and as such represents an ideological break with the postwar concept of a welfare state. As a consequence, collective responsibility for society's vulnerable members has been replaced by a return to liberal values with social policies determined by a market approach to welfare.

The state's role in the provision of welfare has undergone a radical reformulation. This reorientation, established under the Conservative governments of the 1980s and 90s and reconfigured as the Third Way (Blair 1998), under New Labour saw a heightened state retreat from intervention into the economic system (de-regulation) and the re-imposition of moral regulation on social life. Focus turned from the public sector to the private sector, from professional interests to the discipline of the free market and the regulation of the economically redundant underclass by new roles and forms of intervention by social care practitioners.

The reconstruction of health and social services within a mixed economy of care and the rapid construction of a welfare market, exemplified this radical reconceptualisation of the role and responsibilities of the state in relation to health and social welfare. This approach, in line with general central government policies directed at the production of wealth, low taxation and low inflation prioritised the introduction of competition, the reduction of subsidies to consumers and the principle of privatisation, as transitional measures in achieving a conversion to a residual, minimalist role for the state.

The impact of the global economic crisis of the mid-1970s and the adoption

Table 3.1 Changes in the relationship between the individual and the state as indicated by changes in health and social welfare policy in the twentieth and twenty-first centuries

Name	Ideological model	State/individual balance
Welfare state	Collective/socialist	The state takes responsibility for providing health and welfare services available to all. All working people pay into the system through taxes and National Insurance, and services are accessible to all citizens and services such as health, education and welfare (social work and benefits) can be claimed any time they are required. These are generally free. This model enhances equality but may tend to promote a limited range of services as it does not recognise peoples' diversity, strengths and choices.
Mixed economy	Neo-liberal/Third Way	The state shares responsibility with the individual; some facilities such as health and education are still provided through the state system (paid for by taxes) while others, such as social work services, are targeted only at 'the most needy' through a system of eligibility criteria and charges for services. An increasing number of social care services are provided by the private or voluntary sector rather than the state. The role of the 'market' is seen as key in promoting choice and diversity but also as a way to reduce taxes and the role of the state in health and welfare.
Market economy	Coalition Lib/Con	Within this system, the individual is expected to take main responsibility for providing for him or herself. Health and education (and some welfare) services are still available via state provision but the private sector, funded by the individual, is seen as increasingly an option for the better-off in society which leaves state provision under-funded and tends to increase problems of social inequality. This model builds on the previous one by reducing further the role of the state and promotes the idea of social support being provided mainly by the community or the 'Big Society'.

Source: Created by G. Koubel, 2012.

of the 'new right ideologies' following the election of the Conservative government in 1979 together caused the basic assumptions about the principles and feasibility of the welfare state to be questioned. One consequence of this was that the professional aspirations of health and social care workers (Stevenson 1988) became an early victim of the subsequent shift from a welfare state model to a mixed economy of welfare that now characterises UK social services. The 'new right' social policies as implemented throughout the 1980s and early 1990s through various legislative and policy initiatives impacted significantly upon professional practice. This was most notable in the adoption of a North American system of case management, which is discussed in further detail in Chapter 9. This was a system and approach for assessing needs, planning, providing and reviewing the effectiveness of care for people living in the community where the providers of care were highly diverse and fragmented.

The substitution of a welfare market in place of a welfare state was achieved primarily through the break of the state monopoly in health care and the shift in role of local authority social service departments from one of provider to that of enabler or purchaser. Implementation of this policy was introduced throughout the 1980s and early 1990s through a raft of legislative and policy statements (Cunningham and Cunningham 2008). These and the range of other general welfare policies including the Education Reform, Housing and Local Government Finance Acts 1988 provided the framework within which the architecture of the welfare state could be dismantled.

In moving from the welfare state model of collective responsibility to a system that reduced the role of the state and increased the responsibility of the individual, four ideas have been central.

1. In the Production of Welfare Approach, developed by the Personal Social Services Research Unit at the University of Kent (Davies 1986), a framework of general concepts was proposed which gave credence to a number of important presumptions that paved the way for the repudiation and rejection of the welfare state. What this approach achieved was that welfare services could be converted to a number of objectified commodities (the idea that health and social care could be bought and sold like any other consumer goods) that could be measured and exchanged within a market economy.

2. The adoption of a rational management approach to health and social services the achievement of efficiency, economy and effectiveness became a priority (and ultimately the purpose) of services. The language, focus and concern of managers and practitioners in the personal social services shifted with the introduction of and emphasis given to rationality in planning and resourcing, the application of eligibility criteria, targeting and needs led assessments.

3. New roles and skills were introduced within the workforce for commissioning, contracting and care management functions. These included objective and short-term goal setting, review and audit of the levels of service provided and quality improvement within cost constraints with an emphasis on specification and achievement of measurable objectives. Individual responsibility

was controlled by fixed contracts, performance and pay review; the generation of performance indicators for resource inputs were linked to care outputs; resource allocation was linked to demography and need rather than production and capital costs. This was underpinned by the separation of the discrete functions such as management, purchasing, planning, quality control, and the minimum provision of essential core services. These measures all invoked managerial rather than professional criteria and priorities particularly with regard to budgetary control and allocation. The achievement of tangible outcomes dominated the need to demonstrate performance competence and compliance in meeting operational performance targets; specifying and costing input and output measures; monitoring and reporting mechanisms within the workplace and the acceptance of a competence based approach for establishing national occupational standards for social workers.

4. As health and social services patients and clients were re-designated as 'service users' or re-framed as 'consumers' and service purchasers as 'customers' or 'commissioners' the introduction of consumerism within the welfare economy established a presumption that in managing human services organisations formal arrangements for 'institutional representation' could be replaced with more informal approaches to 'looking after' the customer. Satisfying the customer with service and goods rather than allowing them to influence what is available and offering choice for consumers or purchasers from amongst a range of services and service providers, determined naturally by individual's ability to pay, was rationalised as promoting individual autonomy.

These four notions have, since their introduction during the early 1980s, now taken on the status of social facts and appropriated understandings of the need for, purpose and nature of social policy and services in the UK. Their subsequent impact on the construction of the roles and functions of health and social care workers within prevailing policy highlights the vulnerability of the professions to fluctuating ideologies and central and local authority agendas.

Risk, rights, responsibility in society today

Social welfare institutions in the UK since the 1980s have increasingly adopted policies that approach the issues of wealth and poverty in terms of competition for the available resources in a deregulated competitive economic and political environment and as such have largely followed the liberal tradition of the USA of focusing upon individual performance and pathology. Since the 1990s, with the rising incidents of poverty, crime and associated problems of homelessness, single parenthood, truancy, drug abuse and suicide, attention has returned to nineteenth-century forms of moralisation through coercion of the unemployed and in some cases people who could be seen as vulnerable in 'Welfare to Work' and other treatment programmes.

Additionally the large-scale collective systems and institutions of social protection and social assistance, established at the end of the nineteenth century and consolidated within the postwar welfare state are fragmenting, as the better-off exit from the system and adopt private schemes in a society charac-terised by increasing economic and social diversity and inequality. Here the government is no longer able to carry out its traditional role of maintaining social harmony by limiting unrestrained economic growth for the sake of polit-ical stability.

In a high technology rather than a labour intensive industrialised society, structural unemployment leads to a decline in real income for the majority, and unemployment and poverty for a growing minority, with improved conditions only for a small minority. This increased division of society gives rise to socially privileged minorities who are prepared to tolerate the exclusion of those who have been expelled from the labour process. Social integration is replaced by systems integration, and administrative or economic imperatives transform personal relations, services and phases of life into objects of administration or commodities (Braverman 1974).

As risk management and responsibility shifts downwards towards the individ-ual or to the level of private households, so excluded social groups are left dependent upon measures of compulsory inclusion, expert intervention and corrective enforcement. In the face of the rationalisation of society and the encroachment of economic and administrative processes into everyday life, collectively defined rights and responsibilities have been replaced by the impo-sition on the individual of the burden of the entire responsibility for his or her own fate.

Establishing a framework for fair and responsible self-regulation between the state, the market and the community, the legitimacy of which rests upon the government's authority to set limits upon the formal legal entitlements of the state and the private spheres of economic and family life is elusive. Neither New Labour's Third Way nor the current administrations construct of a Big Society have proven to be adequately convincing as such a framework is required to go beyond the limitations of the protective framework of the rule of law, and the liberal tradition of the social contract, in which individuals are transformed into citizens through the possession of rights. Associated with this increased frag-mentation of society is the view of human nature that presupposes:

> a detached, self-sufficient, independent individual, primarily engaged in pursuing his own self-interest; a being who is fundamentally egocentric, living in competition with and in fear of other individuals. (Sevenhuijsen 1988: 12)

Practice in health and social services, wedded as it is, on the one hand, to the objectives of government social policy and, on the other, to the professional ambitions of its practitioners has become subject to the strategic actions of serv-ice managers, generated in response to central government's modernisation policies. This has given rise to tensions and anxieties within service agencies, between the managers of service organisations and the professional practitioners who implement the agency strategies. Today the relationship between risk, rights and responsibility can easily be seen as a matter of what will work most effectively or produce the best impression upon others in the survival or advancement of managing one's own health, marriage, friendships, career and political goals.

At this level the processes of modernisation (Adams 2003) have implied that therapeutic and educational forms of health and social care work intervention are failing as health and social services can no longer claim to be capable of reducing the numbers of or militating against negative social consequences to and from socially excluded individuals and families. The result has been a necessary realignment between the ethical codes and practice interventions of professionals. Managers of social welfare agencies are faced, on the one hand, with the competing demands of their responsibility for the strategic containment of social risks and, on the other, the requirement that they adopt and comply with central government's modernisation agenda. Their response, presented under the rhetoric of improving services, has been to effectively reconstruct our understanding of what constitutes need, who is entitled to receipt of social services and who is responsible for providing care. This has been achieved by delimiting the strategic responsibilities of local authorities to meet the needs of citizens through the application of continuously tightening eligibility criteria (Department of Health 2003).

Similarly health and social service practitioners have become accustomed to the introduction of procedures and criteria for guiding their activities and to the affects of a continuous process of reorganisation of the remaining structures and frameworks of state institutions and public agencies of welfare. Within this context professional interventions are aimed at achieving the transfer out of service provision to a network of providers in the economic sphere under contract to the core organisation. Concerns over social justice are relegated to the arena of law, as matters of legal rather than moral interpretation and judgement (Norrie 1990; Schwehr 1995; Keenan 1997).

━━━━━━━━━━━━━━━━━━━━━━━━━ **CHALLENGE** ━━━━━━━━━━━━━━━━━━━━━━━━━

Consider the following:

■ Who should and who should not be considered as deserving of or entitled to receive health and social services?

■ How should such decisions be made and by whom?

■ How should vulnerable groups, such as children or frail older people should be looked after or cared for when their families and relatives are unable or unwilling to do so?

These are contested areas where different people in society (or people from different cultures) may hold differing views about where the responsibility for the care of vulnerable people lies; and this has varied considerably throughout history. However, responses to these questions will depend not only upon a person's political affiliation but also on their values and beliefs around social justice, risk and the role of the state. These diverse constructions of risks, rights and responsibilities will be explored in greater depth in subsequent chapters.

Conclusion

Most recently the identification, assessment, management and avoidance of risk have become a dominant force in shaping how health and social services respond to these questions. The ways in which professional practitioners have responded to questions of risk, rights and responsibilities has been shaped by the organisations in which they practise with close connections to social policy and its function within the UK political-administrative system of government. Practitioners therefore struggle to maintain good ethical practice in the face of bureaucratic restrictions and procedures which limit rather than liberate creative practice. Nowhere is this more apparent than in the sphere of safeguarding vulnerable people from the risks they may face from their own naïve actions but more particularly from others who may neglect, exploit or abuse them.

Attempts to recapture the credibility and legitimacy of the professions have followed the tragic death of Baby Peter and more sophisticated approaches to risk assessment and management are being identified (Munro 1996), developed (Green and McDermott 2010), and implemented (London Borough of Hackney 2008). In a society that is orientated towards increased liberalisation, matters of risks, rights and responsibilities within the health and social services are increasingly a matter of legal and professional determinations of individual vulnerability and capacity, rather than universal entitlements. However, we should remain aware of the complex and powerful political and psychological forces that shape our understanding of and responses to matters of risk, rights and responsibility.

Today, as uncertainty increases, and where firm foundations and consistent situations are replaced by uncertainty and unpredictability, so norms and values become unstable, our confidence is shaken and the social order rests more on structures of expectations than of knowledge. Melville-Wiseman in Chapter 7 explores the rights, risks and responsibilities involved in building trusting relationships between practitioners and people who use mental health services. Under these conditions trust assumes an important role in shaping and mediating social relations.

> Trust makes it possible to interact on uncertain premises, without firm knowledge, knowing only that it is possible to predict future actions with a certain amount of probability. We do not need trust in certain and constant situations, where confidence prevails and alternatives are unconsidered. However, in unfamiliar, unpredictable and deviant situations we need trust, which implies the acknowledgement of contingent choice, and the responsibility involved in choice. (Holmstom 2007)

References

Adams, A. (2003) *The Modernisation of Social Work Practice and Management in England*. Eichstatt: iSiS Verlag ALBERT Czech Republic.

Barr, N. (1987) *The Economics of the Welfare State*. London: Weidenfeld and Nicolson.

Beck, U. (1992) *Risk Society: Towards a New Modernity*. London: Sage.

Blair, T. (1998) *The Third Way: New Politics for the New Century*. London: Fabian Society.

Blakemore, K. (2003) *Social Policy: An Introduction* (2nd edn). Buckingham: Open University Press.

Braverman, H. (1974) *Labour and Monopoly Capital: The Degradation of Work in the Twentieth Century*. New York: Monthly Review Press.

Burkitt, I. (1997) Social relationships and emotions. *Sociology*, 31(1): 37–55.

Cox, R. H. (1998) The consequences of welfare reform: how conceptions of social rights are changing. *Journal of Social Policy*, 27(1): 1–16.

Cunningham, J. and Cunningham, S. (2008) *Sociology and Social Work* Exeter: Learning Matters.

Davies, B. P. (1986) The production of welfare approach. Discussion Paper 400, Canterbury: PSSRU, University of Kent.

Department of Health (2003) *Fair Access to Care Services*. London: Department of Health.

Donnelly, J. (2003) *Universal and Human Rights: In Theory and Practice*. Ithaca, NY: Cornell University Press.

Douglas, M. (1970) *Natural Symbols: Explorations in Cosmology*. New York: Vintage Books.

Elias, N. (2000) *The Civilising Process* (trans. Edmund Jephcott). Cambridge: Polity Press.

Foucault, M. (1980) *Power / Knowledge Selected Interviews and other Writings, 1972–1977* (ed. Colin Gordon). London: Harvester Press.

Furedi, F. (2008) *Paranoid Parenting*. London: Continuum.

Giddens, A. (1990) *The Consequences of Modernity*. Stanford, CA: Stanford University Press.

Gilbert, L. and Dunn, T. (2009) Person-centred primary care and health promotion. In G. Koubel and H. Bungay (eds), *The Challenge of Person-Centred Care*. Basingstoke: Palgrave Macmillan.

Green, D. and McDermott, F. (2010) Social work from inside and between complex systems: perspectives on person-in-environment for today's social work. *British Journal of Social Work*, 40(8): 2414–30.

HMSO (1942) *Social Insurance and Allied Services*, CMND 6404.

Hobsbawm, E. J. (1994) *The Age of Extremes: The Short Twentieth Century, 1914–1991*. London: Michael Joseph.

Hogg, M. and Abrams, D. (1998) *Social Identifications*. London: Routledge.

Holmstom, S. (2007) Niklas Luhmann: contingency, risk, trust and reflection. *Public Relations Review*, 33: 255–62.

Jacobs, J. (ed.) (1992) *Beveridge 1942–1992*. London: Whiting and Birch.

Keenan, C. (1997) Finding that a child is at risk from sexual abuse: re H (Minors) (Sexual Abuse: Standard of Proof). *Modern Law Review*, 60(6): 857–65.

Keynes J. M. (1936) *The General Theory of Employment, Interest and Money*. Basingstoke: Palgrave Macmillan.

Koubel, G. and Bungay, H. (2009) *The Challenge of Person-Centred Care: An Interprofessional Perspective*. Basingstoke: Palgrave Macmillan.

London Borough of Hackney (2008) *A Difference that Makes a Difference: Clinical Manual, The Role of Clinicians in the Social Work Unit.* Available at: http://www.cityandhackneycamhs.org.uk/wordpress/wp-content/themes/camhs_white/downloads/csc-clinical-manual.pdf

Luhmann, N. (1993) *Risk: A Sociological Theory.* Cambridge: Cambridge University Press.

Luhmann, N. (1996) Complexity, structural contingencies and value conflicts. In P. Heelas, S. Lash and P. Morris (eds), *Detraditionalisation.* Oxford: Blackwell.

Munro, E. (1996) Avoidable and unavoidable mistakes in child protection work. *British Journal of Social Work*, 26(6): 793–808.

Norrie, K. (1990) Resource allocation in health care: the role of the courts. In U. J. Jenson and G. Mooney (eds), *Changing Values in Medical and Health Care Decision Making.* Chichester: John Wiley & Sons.

Offe, C. (1984) *The Contradictions of the Welfare State.* London: Hutchinson.

Offe, C. (1996) *Modernity and the State.* Cambridge: Polity Press.

Perkin, H. (1969) *The Origins of Modern English Society 1790–1880.* London: Routledge & Kegan Paul.

Philp, M. (1979) Notes on a form of knowledge in social work. *Sociological Review*, 27: 183–211.

Powell, M. and Hewitt, M. (2002) *Welfare State and Welfare Change.* Buckingham: Open University.

Schwehr, B. (1995) The legal relevance of resources – or a lack of resources – in community care. *Journal of Social Welfare and Family Law*, 17(2): 179–98.

Sevenhuijsen, S. (1998) *Citizenship and the Ethics of Care.* London: Routledge.

Stevenson, O. (1998) It was more difficult than we thought: a reflection on 50 years of child welfare practice. *Child and Family Social Work*, 3: 153–61.

Tajfel, H. (1981) *Human Groups and Social Categories.* Cambridge: Cambridge University Press.

PART II

Theory in Practice

Managing Risk in a Complex Society

Georgina Koubel and Cheryl Yardley

Introduction

This chapter looks at various ways of conceptualising, assessing and managing risk within society, making links with issues such as risk and dangerousness, risk aversion; models for assessing and understanding the nature of risk in health and social work/care; and the perception of risk by professional groups and the media. The chapter uses scenarios that highlight risk and explores ways in which these may be addressed within the framework of safeguarding both children and vulnerable adults. The application of models of risk analysis to particular scenarios of risk and concern will focus on the professionals' perception of risk, the rights and the responsibilities of various stakeholders and the management of risk in complex situations (Titterton 2005).

While the chapter considers the merits of a range of risk assessment models (including actuarial models, and Brearley) the focus of the chapter is on the level/layers of complexity that includes the changing and dynamic nature of risk that challenging cases entail, therefore requiring a model of risk assessment that can encompass this complexity. The reflective challenges require the reader to look in some detail at two cases which raise issues of risk, safeguarding and protection, one involving a child in the family and another looking at the situation of a disabled person living in the community. The first particularly highlights issues of responsibility and the balance of the rights of the child and the parents, the other focuses more on issues of vulnerability, choice, capacity and human rights. In both cases the legal and ethical frameworks will be analysed for their relevance and usefulness.

This chapter is written by two social workers, one who has worked mainly in the field of children and families and the other who has considerable experience working in Adult Services. If we accept that values and attitudes are formed from a combination of personal experiences, professional values and society's expectations of the way in which professionals carry out the roles and tasks that inform their occupation, then this chapter provides an opportunity to gain insight into similarities and differences in the ways risk, rights and responsibilities can be framed to affect professional intervention depending on the context of that intervention. The conclusion is informed by reference to established work on human rights, models of risk and ethical and legislative frameworks across Britain relevant to child and adult safeguarding.

LEARNING OUTCOMES

By the end of the chapter you should have developed your understanding of:

- The advantages and limits of a number of models of risk assessment

- How the social construction of risk and vulnerability can inform risk assessment and decision making

- The understanding and application of a model of complex risk assessment to different scenarios

- The importance of inter-professional and collaborative working in managing complex and dynamic situations.

There are a number of reflection points to enable readers to consider:

- Their own attitudes to risk, rights and responsibility

- The social construction of risk and vulnerability

- The delicate balance between rights and risks

- The inter-professional nature of accountability, responsibility and collaboration

- The balance between empowerment, choice, rights and safety for service users

- The importance of recognising and acknowledging the perspectives of stakeholders

- Person-centred approaches when working with individuals, families and carers

- The value and limits of policies, procedures and professional knowledge

- Knowledge, skills and values that inform practice and decision making in situations of complexity and change.

→

→

Having looked at the theoretical constructs around rights, risks and responsibilities in the previous chapters, we begin this one by asking you to question yourself about some issues that are relevant to you both personally and professionally.

━━━━━━━━━━━━━ **CHALLENGE** ━━━━━━━━━━━━━

Think about these carefully and honestly and start to analyse how these values and attitudes may inform your practice.

■ What does risk mean to you? What first comes to mind when you think about the notion of risk? Is it a positive or negative sensation?

■ Where do you think your ideas come from? Can you remember your earliest awareness of risk? How do you think these affected you?

■ Would you say your personal attitudes to risk are the same as the ones you would employ in your professional role?

■ How do you think this would affect your decision making in practice?

Beck (1992, 2004) talks of the problems of living in a risk-averse society, and thereby implies that professional practitioners are likely to err on the side of caution when weighing the costs and benefits of a particular course of action. Stanford (2010) addresses the 'moral dilemmas of risk in social work' where she identifies that

> the negative ramifications of this for clients are a core concern of the critical social work risk literature. This literature claims that social work practices actively construct clients as objects of risk to be studied, measured and corrected.

Hazel Kemshall (2010) looks at the question of risk within social work and acknowledges that the concept of risk is neither 'uniform (n)or uncontested'. She explores the notion of different rationalities of risk depending on whether the subject of professional intervention is seen as 'the rational actor' or the 'responsibilised' person. She goes on to explore this further.

> The rational actor is rooted in economic theory that sees risk choices as located in an economic rationality of cost and benefit, and that actors will only make sub-optimal choices if information is poor or incorrect. (2010: 2)

This leads us on think about notions of vulnerability (*No Secrets*, Department of Health 2000) which may be affected by such features as age (too young, too old), disability (too frail, too weak), or mental capacity (irrational, irresponsible, too easily exploited). This suggests that our attitudes towards risk are affected depending on how we assess the ability of the person to undertake the risk. So, for example, a risk that you or I might undertake every day (for example driving to work, taking a night bus) might be assessed as too great a risk for someone who is perceived as vulnerable.

Fear informs the assessment of the social worker, whether it is fear for clients or fear for her/himself, or the fear of being negatively judged by clients, the media or the wider society (Stanford 2010). Often social workers feel they cannot win: if they intervene they are called 'child snatchers' and interfering busybodies; it may therefore not be surprising that social workers are fearful of taking risks when they know if a tragedy occurs, they will be vilified by the press, possibly by their employers and even by their regulatory body. Of course there is also concern that a vulnerable person may be harmed in the process but because of the response by the media and the public there is a deep-seated anxiety about some of the dangerous and risky practices that service users may engage in, and social workers have to find models that can help them identify the risk factors, measure and weigh them in terms of potential outcomes.

The social work risk literature is littered with the suggestion that a defensive approach to social work practice has become typical of social work interventions … However the majority of social workers' actions in this study indicate that they took a stand for their clients. (Stanford 2010)

The principles and process of risk assessment

In the current context of health and social care practice, where the outcomes of decisions have such significant consequences and there is the likelihood of 'blame by media' if mistakes are made, the use of models of risk can be seen as an attempt to make what is essentially uncertain – what Kelly (in O'Hagan 2007) calls an 'informed guess' about the future – appear certain and measurable. Broadhurst *et al.* (2010) suggest that structured risk assessment tools reduce the element of discretion in decision making, and that this can be seen as a significant advantage. A structured tool should reduce subjectivity in the assessment of risk and provide greater clarity to aid decision making. We will use the following case study to consider some of the issues in using risk assessment tools:

CASE STUDY: CONSIDERING RISK FACTORS

Casey is 17 years old. She was brought up by foster carers from the age of 4 due to physical abuse and neglect by her mother and stepfather, but due to her challenging behaviour she moved placement several times. At the age of 14 she absconded from her foster home and spent several months living rough, and during this time began drinking heavily and using heroin. Following an arrest for shoplifting she was returned

➔

➡

to foster care where she revealed that she was 6 months pregnant; she would not disclose the identity of the father. She was moved to a mother and baby foster placement for an assessment and given support to prepare for the birth. Joshua was born 6 weeks prematurely and admitted to the special care unit. Casey visited a few times but informed the nurse that she didn't want to hold him because he was so small and they were concerned at her lack of interest in his care.

On discharge from hospital Joshua and Casey were placed in a mother and baby foster placement but a week later Casey left with Joshua. She was found 2 days later in the home of a known drug dealer when police were called by neighbours due to reports of a baby screaming. Joshua's clothing and nappy had not been changed, he had been sick after Casey had refilled his bottle with cow's milk and he was in significant distress. Casey had used heroin and was unconscious. Joshua was immediately taken into police protection and placed with a foster carer and the local authority commenced care proceedings. Casey returned to foster care but failed to cooperate with the assessment. She attended several contact sessions late or under the influence of alcohol or drugs and asked the contact supervisor to change and feed Joshua. She said that she found it hard to love him and became agitated when he cried. After three weeks she again absconded from the foster placement and could not be found. Joshua was made subject to a Care Order under Section 31 of the Children Act 1989 and placed for adoption.

Casey, now aged 17, has been to see a GP and disclosed that she is 8 months pregnant. She is living with her boyfriend of 10 months, Jon, in a room in the attic of his father's house; he is doing some occasional work for a builder, she was working in a shop but has now lost her job because of the pregnancy. She states that she has not misused drugs or alcohol for at least 18 months and that they are in a stable relationship and hoping to move into their own flat soon because Jon's dad is planning to sell his house and move away; she says that they 'don't get on' as he often drinks. She says that she and Jon are both happy about the baby and ready to be parents, and they have started buying what they need.

=== CHALLENGE ===

■ What would you identify as possible risk factors in this scenario?

■ Which factors would you see as most significant for your assessment?

In weighing up the risks in this scenario, there are a number of possible tools you could use to guide your thinking. There is a wide variation in the tools available and they all rely on some level of human judgement to weigh up the available data. The common distinction between types of risk assessment tool is that they are 'clinical' or 'actuarial' (Munro 2008; Calder 2008; O'Sullivan 2011). Clinical models rely on the judgement of the practitioner, what Munro describes as their 'intuitive appraisal of the range of information gathered' (2008: 66). An example of a model which relies on the professional expertise of

Table 4.1 A grid to assess risk based on Brearley's framework

Background risk factors	Current risk factors	Dangers	Positive factors
Casey's history of abuse and neglect	Short-term relationship	Neglect of the baby's physical and emotional needs	Casey is no longer using drugs and alcohol
Casey's history of drug and alcohol misuse	Lack of stable income and suitable housing	Poor home environment may cause risk of physical harm, e.g. falls, poor hygiene	Casey and Jon are both happy about the baby
Casey's failure to bond with Joshua	Unsuitable housing	Medical problems due to lack of ante-natal care	They are preparing for the birth and have plans to move to more suitable housing
Casey's neglect of Joshua	Lack of family support	Isolation and stress due to lack of support	Casey has now accessed support

the practitioner is that of Brearley (1982). Brearley's model requires practition-ers to identify hazards, strengths and dangers (the feared or undesirable outcome) and differentiates between predisposing or background hazards, and situational or current hazards (O'Sullivan 2011; Titterton 2005).

Applying this type of approach to the above case study, the assessment of some of the risks may resemble the one shown in Table 4.1.

You may have identified other factors. How straightforward is it to distin-guish between background and situational factors? From our own experience of using this model with students, this can be confusing and some factors may appear in both columns, for example with Casey you may consider her lack of engagement with services in the past as a background hazard, while her lack of accessing ante-natal care earlier in her pregnancy can be seen as a situational hazard. We have suggested that her relationship with Jon is 'short term' and that this is a hazard. Others may feel that 10 months, with clear plans for a future together, suggests a relatively stable relationship and would consider this a strength. The other issue identified as a limitation of Brearley's approach is that while it helps to distinguish between factors it does not help with the analy-sis of how likely the 'dangers' are and how the strengths may mitigate against the hazards. The use of columns may lead to what Titterton (2005) suggests is a 'simple totting up' approach, where more factors in one column may influ-ence the overall decision.

> Risk, for Brearley, is thus simply the gap between 'best' and 'worst' outcome, and has nothing to say about the probability of outcomes ... [thus] in many areas of social intervention, decisions pertaining to risk are inextricably tied up with judgments of probability, and the relative likelihood of different patterns or kinds of outcomes. (Parsloe 1999: 21)

Actuarial models are seen as more objective and rely on risk predictors identified through research, and may require the practitioner to assess factors according to a numerical scale. There are considerable overlaps between the two models: clinical models will rely on the practitioners' evidence base of risk factors, drawing both on their experience and on the available research, while actuarial models will still require an element of judgement in scaling factors and assessing the relevance of the present information to the tool. So while actuarial models appear to be more objective and reliable than those models based on clinical judgement, in fact there will still be some inconsistency in how they are used and an element of subjectivity, for example whether a factor is scaled as low, medium or high risk.

All risk assessment tools rely on consideration of a range of risk factors which have been identified either through practice wisdom or research. These factors are considered predictive of future harm; they may include personal factors such as age, gender and disability, family factors such as domestic abuse and parental or spousal alcohol or substance misuse, and environmental factors, such as poor housing and isolation from support. Factors may be static and unchanging, such as background or historical factors, or dynamic, such as family relationships (O'Sullivan 2011). Several actuarial models rely on static factors, for example the Rapid Risk Assessment for Sex Offence Recidivism (RRASOR) tool: the four factors found to have some predictive accuracy were:

1. The number of past sex offence convictions or charges (with additional weight given to sex offence history)

2. Age of the offender is less than 25

3. Offender is unrelated to victim

4. Gender of victim. (Hanson 1997, cited by Kemshall 2001)

An alternative, however, which claims equal success as a predictive tool is the Structured Anchored Clinical Judgement (SACJ) tool, which also considers dynamic factors such as whether the offender had ever married, substance abuse and deviant sexual arousal. There is less consensus among tools used to assess risk of child abuse. The majority of tools are found in the USA; Britain has been 'interested but more hesitant than either the US or Australia in wholeheartedly adopting structured risk assessment instruments' (Saunders and Goddard 1998: 18). However as Munro (2008) highlights, many of these tools have not been empirically validated, and there is a wide variation in the risk factors identified. She raises concern about the cultural sensitivity of risk factors and whether they are equally applicable in all cases. Greenland's (1987) high-risk checklist of factors (as cited by Corby 2006) includes:

- Single parent/separated
- Poverty; unemployed/unskilled worker; inadequate education
- Child under 5 years old
- Premature or low birth weight.

The definition of 'inadequate education' may vary significantly. The impact of factors such as poverty and single parenthood and the stress they will cause depends on the context in which the family is living and the support available to them, and the social and cultural consequences. Taylor (2010) considers a wider range of factors drawn from other authors according to those risk factors in the parent (such as substance misuse, employment and expectations of the child), the child (premature birth, behaviour and disability), family (poverty, housing and attachment) and the environment (social isolation and systems for identifying and managing abuse). Applying these to the case study we can see that there are a high number of parental, family and environmental factors which could be considered risks. Again, though a list such as this may assist in identifying risks, it does not help to consider the interrelationship between risk factors, how risks accumulate over time and which factors may be more significant in any particular case (Saunders and Goddard 1998).

A further difficulty is that the validity of some of the identified risk factors may be questionable, even where they are based on statistics, due to sampling issues. Much research into abuse and neglect is retrospective and carried out on families where abuse has already taken place. Research, for example, highlights that parental alcohol misuse is a significant factor in instances of child abuse because 40 per cent of children subject to a child protection plan have a parent who abuses alcohol (Corby 2006). This research is based on a limited population – those children who have been identified as suffering or at risk of suffering harm, were referred to social services and met the criteria for a child protection conference. An alternative perspective could come from research into the number of parents in the UK who drink alcohol to excess and do not abuse their children. Stevens and Hassett (2007) suggest that many tools assume a clear causal link between factors and consequences and lead to a linear approach to decision making which ignores the complexity of assessment.

The absence or lack of knowledge about risk factors may lead to complacency in assessment, while the presence of one factor on the list may significantly impact on the assessment; Saunders and Goddard (1998) suggest that risk factors can be spurious or misleading, especially for inexperienced workers.

=== **CHALLENGE** ===

Consider the case study again:

- What information is missing?
- How important is it that you don't know what you don't know?

As Munro (2008) points out having too much information can be over-whelming and confuse an assessment. In this case much of the present informa-tion is regarding historical factors and it will be important to take into account contextual changes, such as her age, her relationship and information about her partner. Taylor's (2010) risk factors in the child which may have been consid-ered significant in assessing the risk to Joshua, such as his prematurity, are unknown for the unborn baby, and Casey's ability to bond with the baby cannot be predicted. The social worker carrying out an assessment would be mindful of their legal responsibilities towards the unborn baby and the princi-ple that the 'welfare of the child is paramount' (Children Act 1989, s. 1), yet in a case such as this making the best decision in the welfare of the child is not straightforward.

Given the identified risk factors and the consequences of a 'wrong' decision, the practitioner may be led to take what could be seen as a low risk decision and ensure supervision of Casey with the baby and even possibly separation. But is this a low risk decision? A practitioner may be aware of the extensive body of research into the poorer outcomes of children who are looked after by the state and also aware of statutory legal responsibilities towards Casey, who is 17 and a care leaver, and her rights as a parent. The 'rule of optimism' would allow that Casey has matured and that she has changed, but practitioners may be influ-enced by the very significant level of risk to which she exposed Joshua and their emotions about this incident may lead them to consider that the negative outcomes of allowing her to care for the new baby unsupervised outweigh any other outcomes. To assist in assessing risk Stevens and Hassett (2007: 136) propose using complexity theory as this can be more dynamic; rather than focusing on cause and effect it seeks 'to understand the interaction between factors'. Their model requires consideration of a range of factors and in partic-ular how they may impact on each other. The practitioner works through a series of stages to identify risks and how these could be reduced:

1. The impact and likelihood of different risks

2. Spatial analysis – the effect of space, place and time

3. Quantitative and qualitative statements of risk

4. Control mechanisms.

In this case, the practitioner may consider the risk of Casey neglecting her baby and consider that while the potential impact of this would be severe, the likelihood is currently low. However, if she were to resume drug or alcohol misuse this would increase. They would consider the impact on Casey of her living conditions and the stress of the potential move and poor relationship with Jon's father, and consider statements such as:

■ The greatest risks are that the baby's physical needs will be neglected lead-ing to significant health and developmental problems

- The risks are increased in the current home particularly at times when Jon is at work and his father has been drinking and Casey feels under stress and without support

- The risks are reduced when Jon is present and able to support Casey in caring for the baby

- The actions that are essential to reduce the risks are that Jon and Casey are rehoused, and that they receive parenting advice and professional support.

The complexity model highlights that assessments of risk cannot be predictive and that many tools lead to a false sense of security. Using such a model in this case would allow the practitioner to consider a wider range of factors and potential outcomes and in particular to clearly focus on the actions which may reduce the risks, leading to a more flexible and less risk-averse approach to risk (Stevens and Hassett 2007).

CASE STUDY: RISK, CHOICE AND EMPOWERMENT

Androulla is a 25-year-old woman who has lived all her life with her mother, Mrs Kyriakou who is now 70. Mrs Kyriakou migrated with her family to England over 30 years ago from Cyprus. Quite recently, following the death of her husband, Mrs Kyriakou moved from a bungalow in North London and now lives with Androulla in a spacious two-bedroomed flat in a private housing block in a small town in a semi-rural area. Androulla has moderate learning disabilities and does not speak very clearly but has strong opinions and is able to make them known. Mrs Kyriakou and her husband always looked after Androulla who requires some help and supervision with activities of daily living. Mrs Kyriakou says that since her husband died she was finding the care of Androulla too much on her own, so moved to be nearer Androulla's sister Alexandra and her husband Tomas and their two children. Alexandra is very busy with her own family life and says she cannot offer much help to her mother and Androulla but Tomas, who takes Androulla to the Day Centre and picks her up at the end of the day, says that Androulla sometimes has visits from friends when her mother is not at home. One of these friends is Duncan, aged 45, who works at the Day Centre and who lives quite near to Androulla.

Androulla has become extremely fond of Duncan, a man who has minor physical and learning disabilities and is employed part-time as a support worker at the Centre. The Centre Manager, Delia Small, tells you that she has been told by other people who attend the Centre that Duncan and Androulla have been seen hugging and kissing. Delia has expressed considerable concern about how this may affect the reputation of the Day Centre and says she will 'have a word' with Duncan and Androulla. Duncan says they are just friends but Androulla claims they are in love and want to get married. Duncan says he goes over to see Androulla one or two evenings a week as Mrs Kyriakou often goes out to play cards and have a drink with her friends within the

→

→

block, and Androulla doesn't like to be left alone. However, Duncan has been seen chatting with Sally Vernon, the practice nurse who comes regularly to the Centre to check on the medical needs of the people who attend. She also gives advice about contraception. Both Alexandra and Mrs Kyriakou have expressed concerns that Duncan is placing Androulla at risk by visiting her at home. Mrs Kyriakou says that in her country her beliefs mean there would be no possibility of allowing this kind of contact between members of the opposite sex among people with disabilities, and that it is the responsibility of the Day Centre manager to forbid Duncan from visiting Androulla to ensure that Androulla is not put in a position where she could be sexually exploited.

CHALLENGE

What are your initial thoughts about what might be going on in this case?

■ What are the risks that come to your mind?

■ What issues are you aware of in terms of the rights of the various parties involved?

■ Whose responsibility is it to do what?

Which of these facts would concern you most? Would there be any differences between your personal and professional concerns?

■ The fact that Duncan is alone with Androulla outside the Centre without parental (or other) supervision

■ The fact that he has been seen kissing and hugging Androulla – is this appropriate for a member of staff? Is he telling the truth and are people reading too much into this?

■ The risk of a sexual relationship and concomitant risks around pregnancy and sexually transmitted diseases?

■ The risk to the reputation of the Day Centre or to Androulla herself?

■ Something else?

Whose rights are we talking about here and what rights are relevant?

■ As an adult Androulla has a right to have her wishes and choices respected. One of the main differences between the legislation that covers the welfare of children and that of adults is that with children the local authority can intervene in the child's best interest even if the child says that they do not wish for intervention. With adults, there is no legislative power or duty to intervene against the person's wishes unless there is proof that the adult is incapacitated and therefore unable to make the decision. This requires an assessment under the Mental Capacity Act 2005, but unless Androulla cannot understand the concepts involved, 'fundamentally, adults are presumed to have mental capacity and the right to make their own decisions' (Mantell and Scragg 2008: 85).

■ If mental capacity is assumed for adults and it cannot be proved that Androulla is incapable of making a decision under the Mental Capacity Act, then she has rights as an adult to make her own decisions and choices. Under the Human Rights Act 1998, she has a number of rights which she shares with all other adults, such as the right to freedom of expression (Article 11), the right to respect for private and family life (Article 8), the right to marry or form a civil partnership (Article 12) and under Article 14 the right not to be discriminated against in respect of these rights and freedoms.

■ However, Androulla also has a right as a vulnerable adult not to be subjected to abuse (*No Secrets*, Department of Health 2000) and safeguarding vulnerable adults should concern everyone.

■ As Androulla is an adult, Mrs Kyriakou is not expected by law to carry out parental rights and responsibilities in the same way she would as if Androulla were a child. However, if it can be proved that Androulla is not capable of understanding the consequences of her decisions, this raises the matter of who should have the responsibility for making decisions on her behalf and *in her best interests*.

■ Duncan also has some rights in this situation. He is being accused of acting at the very least inappropriately and possibly with criminal intent towards Androulla. It may not be possible to determine the extent of his complicity with Androulla; their relationship may indeed be just a friendly one but also it is possible that a criminal act is being carried out under the Sexual Offences Act 2003, in which case the police may need to be involved. As someone who works at the Day Centre that Androulla attends, Duncan has professional responsibilities under this Act not to engage in a sexual relationship with Androulla *whether she consents or not*. However, Duncan's human rights to a fair trial (Article 6) could also be compromised if the matter is not addressed more directly.

■ There may also be particular cultural aspects to this case that need to be considered. While it may be reasonable to consider Mrs Kyriakou's views which may, as she claims, stem from her cultural background, this may have to be overridden by consideration of Androulla's human rights to family and private life. This is important because it requires the practitioner to balance *competing rights* within the context of anti-discriminatory practice (Thompson 2006). Are Androulla's rights as a disabled person more important than Mrs Kyriakou's rights to have her cultural and possibly religious views taken into account? How might this affect the relationships involved?

■ Whatever your personal, human or moral response to the situation you have been hearing about, as a practitioner you have a responsibility to weigh up the risks against the rights of the various parties. In this case it seems that Androulla has a right to have any kind of relationship she likes with anyone she likes (inasmuch as we all are) unless the professionals involved can prove that she is not capable of understanding the consequences of her decision to do so. Even though Androulla may be defined under the No Secrets guidance (2000) as a vulnerable adult who needs services under the National Health Services and Community Care Act 1990, this does not automatically mean that she is unable to understand and make her own decisions. As previously stated, the assumption of autonomy is critical when working with adults. However, it does appear that the estimation of Androulla's capacity is relevant to any decisions and interventions that may be carried out in respect of the information that has been received in this situation. This will require a closer look at the Mental Capacity Act.

Principles to guide decision making under the Mental Capacity Act 2005

- A person must be assumed to have capacity unless it is established that he does not (s. 1(2)).

- A person is not to be treated as unable to make a decision unless all practicable steps to help him do so have been taken without success (s. 1(3)).

- A person is not to be treated as unable to make a decision merely because he makes an unwise decision (s. 1(4))

- An act done, or a decision made for or on behalf of a person who lacks capacity must be done in his best interests (s. 1(5)).

The determination of (in)capacity

- There are two stages: establishing impairment or disturbance of mind, and a resulting inability to make the decision.

- A lack of capacity cannot be established merely by reference to a person's age or appearance, or a condition of his, or an aspect of his behaviour, which might lead others to make unjustified assumptions about his capacity. These rules out the risk of stereotyping and links with a social model of vulnerability (Martin 2007).

- A person is unable to make a decision for himself if he is unable:
  - ☐ to understand the information relevant to the decision
  - ☐ to retain the information
  - ☐ to use or weigh that information as part of the process of making the decision, or
  - ☐ unable to communicate that decision (e.g. in a coma or locked-in state).

Risk, rights and responsibilities in safeguarding vulnerable adults

Whether or not it is determined that Androulla has the capacity and right to make her own decisions, the question of whether she is being abused still needs to be considered. Decision making is likely to involve careful deliberation among professionals, service users and other stakeholders in order to achieve an appropriate balance between concerns and worries and the choices and wishes of individuals which others may feel place them at further risk.

> Adult abuse cases present complex practice and ethical issues for professionals. Central to these is the debate about 'protection versus autonomy'.
> (Brammer 2010: 496)

As a practitioner from any profession within health and social care, you may be required to make judgements and have opinions about whether abuse has taken place. You need to familiarise yourself with whatever policies and procedures are available within your particular area of practice but it is vital to remember that safeguarding, whether of adults or children, is never simply a procedural matter. The task may fall to you to ensure the individual(s) involved are placed at the centre of any safeguarding process and their voice, choices, wishes and rights are not lost in the anxiety about professional responsibility to assess and contain any risks (Koubel and Bungay 2009). While it is extremely unlikely that you would be left alone to determine the seriousness and risk in a complex situation, you may be a vital witness or hold essential information that will contribute to the decision-making process.

Using a complexity model of risk, you would consider:

- What are the key areas of risk?

- Who is at risk from whom?

- When are these risks most apparent?

- How do these risks potentially conflict with rights, choices and values?

- Who has the responsibility to do what in order to minimise and manage the risks?

One of the factors that may affect the way that individuals and practitioners would respond to a situation like that of Duncan and Androulla's is the model not just of risk that you employ but your own construction of the rights and responsibilities of the various parties involved. Those, like Alexandra and Mrs Kyriakou, who appear to equate disability with inevitable vulnerability and the need for Androulla to be protected from certain life experiences may well feel they are acting *in her best interests* by insisting that she and Duncan be forbidden to meet alone as they perceive that her disability may place her at risk. However, a social model of vulnerability that locates risk in the environment rather than in the severity of the impairment of the individual is likely to take a different construction of Androulla's rights and options, including her right as an autonomous adult to make her own decisions and choices.

While Delia Small has a responsibility as his employer to ensure that under the Protection of Vulnerable Groups Act 2006, Duncan does not engage in inappropriate behaviour with any individual who attends the Centre and a duty of care to Androulla to ensure she is not abused or exploited (Association of Directors of Social Services 2005), it is perhaps more difficult to define their responsibility towards Duncan and Androulla in relation to any consensual personal relationship that might develop between them, particularly if either or both of them were to decide to leave the Centre so that they could continue their relationship. While this could be seen as problematic for the accountability of practitioners, it is also possible to look at this relationship in a positive light with the social worker or other practitioners taking on a supportive, proactive or advocacy role based on the principles and values that inform their professional codes of ethics.

However, under a culture of fear (Furedi 2002) there may well be concerns by both the family and Delia Small about how other people in the community and possibly the local or national media would react should the relationship develop to the point where this challenged the social norms of society which may regard the relationship as unacceptable. There could be concerns for the reputation of the Day Centre in terms of whether it is effectively monitoring and safeguarding vulnerable service users, and potentially Androulla herself could be compromised within her culture (and the wider culture) for 'being allowed' to engage in a sexual relationship. One of the most worrying aspects of this situation is the very real risk that Mrs Kyriakou and her family may collaborate with the staff at the Day Centre to develop strategies that will obstruct the relationship between the two individuals concerned, using the respective power and authority they hold over Duncan and Androulla (Thompson 2007) to ensure no relationship develops, thus disregarding their rights and wishes in the name of protection from risk.

Risk management

An alternative way of considering the seemingly irreconcilable views being expressed here is by looking differently at the process of risk assessment and risk management.

As Hothersall and Maas-Lowit (2010) highlight, in comparison to the swathes of material written about risk assessment, the question of risk management has received comparatively little interest. One of the key features of positive risk assessment which inevitably includes an element of risk management is the importance of focusing on the benefits, advantages and opportunities of any course of action as well as addressing areas of risk, concern and potential harm. This means that the risk management plan should be constructed in order to work towards promoting the best likelihood of benefits or positive outcomes while doing what needs to be done to minimise the risk of harmful or negative possibilities (Titterton 2005).

The basic elements involved in risk management include the following:

- Risk management begins from the premise that risk cannot be eliminated, but if the risk is appropriately managed it can reduce the impact of any harm
- Interventions must be proportionate to the degree of perceived risk
- Risk management necessarily involves monitoring role
- If the person(s) concerned is actively engaged with the process, this can be seen as a factor that would reduce risks whereas non-compliance might suggest there are in fact more risks to worry about. (Hothersall and Maas-Lowit 2010: 34)

This model therefore emphasises the importance of engaging all of the stakeholders actively in the discussion and management of the situation. The employment of collaborative practice (Quinney 2006) can provide a model whereby the views and perspectives of all interested parties – including Mrs Kyriakou, Androulla, Duncan, Delia Small, the social worker and any other practitioners such as the practice nurse who attends the Centre – can be explored with a view to establishing the roles and contributions that each could offer to a plan that promotes benefits and supports choices but also plans for managing risks that might arise. By focusing on the benefits and opportunities for Androulla, while also recognising the responsibilities and pressures Mrs Kyriakou has taken on in respect of her daughter over the years, it may be possible to change Mrs Kyriakou's perspective and help her to see how she can help to support Androulla in her move – slowly and gradually – towards independence, while also recognising that Mrs Kyriakou may have her own wishes and concerns about her role as her daughter's carer, and also about her own issues as an older woman coping with loss and change (Currer 2007).

Conclusion

Looking at different models of risk assessment and risk management can help to understand the diverse perspectives – both personal and professional – that may be involved when managing complex and dynamic situations where risks have been identified. Simple, actuarial models of risk assessment may be of assistance when matters are comparatively straightforward. However, the reality of practice means that such situations are often fluid and changeable so that more complex ways of understanding, assessing and managing risk are more usually appropriate. With adults in particular there is very often a tension between the rights, wishes and autonomy of the individual and the risks and concerns that are perceived by others. In these cases, it is clear that practitioners have to have a working understanding of the kinds of rights that have to be taken into account as well as the legislation and policies that can either help to promote individual rights or, in cases where capacity is an issue or where abuse is suspected, that can help to protect and safeguard the individual(s) concerned.

Valuing People (Department of Health 2001) and *Valuing People Now* (Department of Health 2009) rightly emphasise the importance of choice and autonomy for adults with learning disabilities. A further level of complexity arises, however, when an adult may be deemed to be vulnerable even though they do have capacity to make decisions. With children there is a well-established procedural framework which guides the social worker and other practitioners in their interventions with children at risk. No assessment of risk can be completed without reflecting the values and attitudes of the practitioners who are carrying out the assessment but there is legislation and statutory guidance to frame and support the decision-making process. There may be tensions between the rights and responsibilities of the parents and the risks their behaviour presents to children but legally there is a clear rule that 'the needs of the child must be paramount', and if there is evidence of significant harm, the child may be removed from a dangerous or risky situation.

However, when working with adults who may be perceived as vulnerable, or who are seen by others as in need of care and protection, there may be no absolute legal right, or indeed any wish, to remove an individual from a risky situation if she or he has the capacity to make an autonomous decision to remain there. Policies and procedures, professional Codes of Ethics and the outcomes of Serious Case Reviews provide some with an essential guidance as to the conduct expected from practitioners involved with safeguarding vulnerable adults, but the ways in which different stakeholders construct matters of risk and vulnerability, and how they understand the balance between rights and risks and the responsibilities of themselves and other professionals will all affect the outcome. This may be in a way that is dynamic and conducive to collaborative practice with colleagues and carers as well as service users. It is at this stage that the knowledge, skills and values of all the relevant parties need to be collated to try to establish the best possible plan to assess, manage and if possible minimise and monitor the risks that are raising concerns without unnecessarily limiting, oppressing or disempowering service user(s) whose views, rights and wishes should be firmly anchored at the heart of the process.

References

Association of Directors of Social Services (2005) *Safeguarding Adults: A National Framework of Standards for Good Practice in Adult Protection Work*. London: ADSS.

Beck, U. (1992, 2004) *Risk Society: Towards a New Modernity*. London: Sage.

Brammer, A. (2010) *Social Work Law* (3rd edn). Harlow: Pearson.

Brearley, P. C. (1982) *Risk in Social Work*. London: Routledge and Kegan Paul.

Broadhurst, K., Hall, C., Wastell, D., White, S. and Pithouse, A. (2010) Risk, instrumentalism and the humane project in social work: identifying the informal logics of risk management in children's statutory services, *British Journal of Social Work*, 40(4): 1046–64.

Calder, M. (ed.) (2008) *Contemporary Risk Assessment in Safeguarding Children*. Lyme Regis: Russell House.

Corby, B. (2006) *Child Abuse: Towards a Knowledge Base* (3rd edn). Maidenhead: Open University Press.

Currer, C. (2007) *Loss and Social Work*. Exeter: Learning Matters.

Department of Health (2000) *No Secrets*. London: Department of Health.

Department of Health (2001) *Valuing People*. London: HMSO.

Department of Health (2009) *Valuing People Now*. London: HMSO.

Furedi, F. (2002) *Culture of Fear*. London: Continuum.

Hothersall, S. J. and Maas-Lowit, M. (2010) *Need, Risk and Protection in Social Work*. Exeter: Learning Matters.

Kemshall, H. (2001) *Risk Assessment and Management of Known Sexual and Violent Offenders: A Review of Current Issues*, Police Research Series: Paper 140. London: Home Office.

Kemshall, H. (2002) *Risk, Social Policy and Welfare*. Buckingham: Open University Press.

Kemshall, H. (2010) Risk rationalities in contemporary social work policy and practice. *British Journal of Social Work* 4 January.

Koubel, G. and Bungay, H. (2009) *The Challenge of Person-Centred Care: An Interprofessional Perspective*. Basingstoke: Palgrave Macmillan.

Mantell, A. and Scragg, T. (eds) (2008) *Safeguarding Adults in Social Work*. Exeter: Learning Matters.

Martin, J. (2007) *Safeguarding Adults*. Lyme Regis: Russell House.

Munro, E. (2008) *Effective Child Protection* (2nd edn). London: Sage.

O'Hagan, K. (ed.) (2007) *Competence in Social Work Practice* (2nd edn). London: Jessica Kingsley.

O'Sullivan, T. (2011) *Decision Making in Social Work* (2nd edn). Basingstoke: Palgrave Macmillan.

Parsloe, P. (ed.) (1999) *Risk Assessment in Social Work and Social Care*. London: Jessica Kingsley.

Quinney, A. (2006) *Collaborative Practice in Social Work*. Exeter: Learning Matters.

Saunders, B. and Goddard, C. (1998) *A Critique of Structured Risk Assessment Procedures: Instruments of Abuse?* Australian Childhood Foundation and the National Research Centre for the Prevention of Child Abuse at Monash Universty, Melbourne.

Stanford, S. (2010) 'Speaking back' to fear: responding to the moral dilemmas of risk in social work practice. *British Journal of Social Work*, 40(4): 1065–80.

Stevens, I. and Hassett, P. (2007) Applying complexity theory to risk in child protection practice. *Childhood*, 14(1): 129–46.

Taylor, B. (2010) *Professional Decision Making in Social Work*. Exeter: Learning Matters.

Thompson, N. (2006) *Anti Discriminatory Practice* (4th edn). Basingstoke: Palgrave Macmillan.

Thompson, N. (2007) *Power and Empowerment*. Lyme Regis: Russell House.

Titterton, M: (2005) *Risk and Risk Taking in Health and Social Care*. London: Jessica Kingsley.

Upholding the Rights of People with Profound Intellectual and Multiple Disabilities

Andy Nazarjuk and Cathy Bernal

Introduction

In 2009, the Joint Committee of the House of Lords and House of Commons on Human Rights noted that adults with learning disabilities are 'particularly vulnerable' to abuse of their rights; it was further stated that within this group, those with profound disabilities are especially at risk (Joint Committee of the House of Lords and the House of Commons 2009). To many agencies and individuals supporting people with such extensive difficulties this was no revelation (e.g. Hogg, in Pawlyn and Carnaby 2009; Department of Health 2009; Mansell 2010). This group of individuals are at significantly greater risk than those with less complex disabilities as a result of ignorance, prejudice and discrimination (Department of Health 2008; Emerson and Baines 2010), factors that contribute directly to the generally poor outcomes of health care treatment for all people with learning disabilities. Furthermore, it is widely acknowledged that beyond the limited confines of the health care setting, people with profound intellectual and multiple disabilities are widely excluded from society, and that concerted and collaborative action is required to remedy this (e.g. Dawkins 2009; Mansell 2010).

LEARNING OUTCOMES

This chapter explores the complexities surrounding the rights, risks and responsibilities concerning profoundly disabled individuals. By the end of the chapter you should have developed your understanding of:

■ The rights of people with profound intellectual and multiple disabilities, the historical abuse of these rights and the contemporary challenges involved in meeting them

■ The risks to which the identified client group are commonly exposed

■ The approaches that support the social inclusion and upholding of the rights of people with profound and complex disabilities.

In advance of the discussion concerning people with profound intellectual and multiple disabilities, it is helpful to define this population; however, this is not aided by the labels that are used to categorise people. Whilst the World Health Organisation (1993) refers to 'profound learning disability', a recent UK publication (Pawlyn and Carnaby 2009) prefers 'profound intellectual and multiple disabilities', a high profile professional network in the UK (PMLD Network, no date) also refers to 'people with profound and multiple learning disabilities', and the International Association for the Scientific Study of Intellectual Disabilities (IASSID) opts more simply for 'profound multiple disabilities' (IASSID, no date). In response to changing transatlantic preference, the term used here will be 'profound intellectual and multiple disabilities' (PIMD).

CHALLENGE

Describe what you understand by the term 'profound intellectual and multiple disabilities'. It may help to think about how you think such a condition may affect an individual in their day-to-day life. Record your ideas in the form of a spider diagram, that is, write the term 'profound intellectual and multiple disabilities' in the middle of a blank piece of paper and draw lines out to your associated ideas.

It is likely that you have generated a variety of different characteristics related to your definition of PIMD. Your spider diagram may include such things as limited communication skills, limited understanding, difficulty in learning, needing help with everyday tasks, lack of opportunity, difficult behaviour and physical disability – these are common things people think of. However, it is important to recognise that a definition or label has the potential to influence how you think about and how you might interact with a person. Definitions by nature are generic and frequently deficit based capturing only the common characteristics of a particular condition and particularly things a person cannot do. They do not always describe other qualities that define the individual as a person with a unique personality, tastes, interests and skills. Before we go on to explore this further, return to your spider diagram and check to see if your definition includes personal qualities as well as deficits.

The PMLD network (PMLD Network, no date) describes their client group as having in common a *profound learning disability*, but in addition a range of other impairments such as sensory difficulties, complex health needs, or mental ill health. All such affected individuals will have great difficulty in communicating, and all will require intense support with their activities of daily living. Whilst acknowledging that reference to intelligence level alone is problematic (McClimens and Richardson 2010), the reader may also like to be aware that the World Health Organisation (1993) defines a profound learning disability as involving an IQ of less than 30, and the American Psychiatric Association (APA) as one of between 20 and 25 (APA 2000). IASSID in this context refers to people 'with such profound cognitive disabilities that no existing standardized tests are applicable for a valid estimation of their level of intellectual capacity and who often possess profound neuromotor dysfunctions' (IASSID, no date). Mansell (2010) noted that individuals thus affected may only use non-verbal means of communication, and show limited evidence of intention, but are nevertheless capable of developing personality and creating meaningful relationships with others (see also Mencap 2006a).

CASE STUDY

Asha is 19 years old, and has been described by her GP as having 'profound learning disabilities', caused by anoxia (oxygen deprivation) at birth. Asha lacks voluntary movement in all four limbs, uses a wheelchair and communicates solely by non-verbal sounds and facial expression. It is not clear whether she intends to convey meaning by these means, or whether they are involuntary. She does not make eye contact with those around her, possibly on account of a suspected visual defect. She is doubly incontinent and fully reliant on her devoted family for all aspects of physical care. This does not include feeding in a conventional sense, as she has had a PEG (percutaneous endoscopic gastrostomy – a feeding tube) inserted some years ago due to swallowing difficulties. She continues to live at home at the request of her parents, and attends a local day service for a few hours a week. People who know Asha communicate with her using touch, facial expression and simple language, though opinion differs as to how much of the latter – if any – she understands. She has been noted to respond positively to music, but as yet this potential has not been developed into a more formal means of communication.

CHALLENGE

◼ Why do you think it is that people like Asha are more likely to be socially excluded?

◼ Do labels, such as those discussed above, contribute to this likelihood? Or are labels necessary for professionals and service users?

A brief history of rights of people with PIMD

Towards the latter part of the nineteenth century and during most of the twentieth century people with PIMD were institutionalised; this was a form of care which incarcerated and segregated a wide range of people considered to be 'mentally defective' under the Mental Deficiency Act 1913 (Race 2002). Under this Act mental deficiency was defined as 'a condition of arrested or incomplete development of mind occurring before the age of 18 years, whether due to inherent causes or induced by injury or disease. It defined four classes of mental defective – idiots, imbeciles, feeble minded and moral defective (Heaton-Ward 1978). Later, under the Mental Health Act 1959, people like Asha were legally defined as demonstrating *severe subnormality* or *subnormality* or were less formally described as being *mentally handicapped* (Heaton-Ward 1978). The places where people were incarcerated and institutionalised were large Victorian asylums or subnormality hospitals which were home to thousands of people and commonly geographically isolated. Together with the process of institutionalisation which denied people their freedom and human rights the language used to describe people served to further dehumanise them. The above terms by today's standards are considered derogatory but their meaning was equally derogatory even when originally introduced, and contributed to the way in which these people were treated.

════════════ **CHALLENGE** ════════════

Before we explore further the historical aspects of the care of people with PIMD consider why you think it is important to know about the history of care provision for this group of people.

■ What difference might this make to the quality of care provided by contemporary health and social care services?

■ How may historical accounts and practices contribute to the formation of our attitudes and behaviour towards people with PIMD?

Attitudes often tend to be negative, based on the notion that people with PIMD are of less human value than other people. More importantly our understanding of the inadequacy and dehumanising processes of large-scale institutionalisation has had an impact on the way contemporary services are provided. Modern residential services, for example, tend to be in ordinary housing, modelled on smaller family units, and there are opportunities for people to have access to personalised funding for their care. Whereas a few decades ago Asha might have been moved into an institution at an early age (regardless of her parents' wishes), today she is supported in the family home, where her parents and siblings are able to purchase the care she needs by means of an individual budget.

Historically the policy of institutionalisation was at its height throughout the first half of the twentieth century, supported by legislation that worked against people's rights and frequently secured their long-term detention (Mental Deficiency Acts 1913, 1927); even the most able people found themselves incarcerated and unable to leave. For example, Joseph 'Joey' Deacon was a patient for over 50 years in St Lawrence's Mental Subnormality Hospital in Caterham Surrey. Deacon suffered from severe cerebral palsy which meant he could not walk, had no obvious intelligible speech and was considered to be mentally subnormal; when in fact he was of normal intelligence (Ellis 1982). Joey was perhaps fortunate to have three close friends in St Lawrence's, one of whom was able to understand him, and together the four men wrote and published a biography of Joey's life in 1974 (Deacon 1974). However, although this represented a significant achievement, it did not eradicate the fact that Joey, because of his disability, and the way that society responded to it, spent the majority of his life excluded from society.

Morris (1969), describing institutions, stated that the 'subnormality' hospitals were more like prisons than general hospitals, and that unlike inmates of prisons most people admitted to subnormality hospitals once admitted never leave.

Further examination of this form of care, particularly in respect of people with profound intellectual and multiple disabilities, exposes a lack of information and silence about their lives. This is unsurprising as this group of people are the *least* likely to be able to *easily* express or communicate their views and opinions to others because of the profound nature of their conditions. The very nature of the condition means that people with this level of impairment are without a personal voice and reliant on others to anticipate or interpret their preferences and needs. Unlike Joey many institutionalised people with PIMD would indeed have been *without a voice* as a result of their profound intellectual impairment. They too were at the mercy of those who cared for them and, as described by Ryan and Thomas (1987), were objectified and treated as less than human.

There are stories written by researchers, reporters and nurses describing the lives of people with PIMD in long-stay institutions. Stories have also been captured in films such as *Silent Minority* (1981) which shows the neglectful conditions found in two UK hospitals for the 'mentally handicapped', and in imagery such as in *Christmas in Purgatory* where Dr Burton Blatt and photographer Fred Kaplan, during their visits of the 'back' wards of five American eastern state institutions, took photographs of the terrible conditions with a hidden camera (Blatt and Kaplan 1974) and a photographic collection of female institutionalised patients by Arbus (1995). These records allow future generations to witness the plight and vulnerability of people with PIMD. Few authors have also told stories of their personal experiences of visiting long-stay institutions (Morris 1969; Ryan and Thomas 1987; Bogdan and Taylor 1994), and leave a testimony of the atrocious standards of care particularly for people with PIMD during that period. Bogdan and Taylor, for example, describe the terrible conditions found on wards where the stench of urine and faeces was overwhelming, and Thomas in his reflections describes the degrading and neglectful circumstances people found themselves in.

Some may perceive these to be extreme examples of institutional life and argue that the conditions of institutional care were exaggerated and unbalanced (Allen 2009). Allen, challenging the negative view of institutional care, makes reference to the kindness of many nurses who dedicated their lives to the care of the 'subnormal' or 'mentally handicapped'. Our personal experience would support this but equally we would argue that the experience of the institutionalised patient was not that of a family life, but one of an institutional regime which for the very vulnerable could be harsh and impersonal. The dedicated nurses who cared for these patients could themselves leave the institution returning to their families on the outside – but the 'patients' did not have this choice, and were at the mercy of the variety of attitudes held by the different staff caring for them.

The documentary on *Silent Minority* (ITN 1981) remains one of the most powerful ethnographic records of institutional lives. A sense of the lives of people in long-stay institutions is illustrated by this quotation from *Silent Minority* by Bob Saunders, a patient of 35 years in St Lawrence's Hospital, who was narrating parts of the film, 'a lot of the poor souls don't know their money, don't know how to read, don't know how to write'. Furthermore, one of the male high dependency wards featured in the film shows how the more able bodied and 'high grade' patients were used as unpaid nurses looking after the more helpless patients. The footage shows that there was not enough staff to look after people so the hospital relied on the more able patients. This was accepted policy and practice and institutions were designed to run in this way – minimally staffed with a range of patients where the more able worked to help run the institution.

> An institution which takes all types of patients is economical because the high grade patients do the work and make everything necessary, not only for themselves, but also for the lower grade … (Wood Report 1929, cited in Race 2002: 32)

As a result the so-called 'lower grade' patient was at the mercy of others, vulnerable and at risk of abuse or neglect. It seems ironic that today carers cannot work with this client group unless they have undergone a number of checks to establish their good character and ability to undertake such a role.

Silent Minority also showed the experience of Terry Green, a 50-year-old patient described as a 'baby', and 'for want of a politer word a *vegetable*', who was perceived as less than human and treated as such. Terry used a wheelchair and could manoeuvre himself about by moving the wheels, despite this the chair he was provided with had such small wheels he could not reach them and so he was denied this freedom and independence; therefore because of his dependency on others who failed to consider his abilities he was denied this right. The language used to describe Terry Green and the language used by Heaton-Ward and Wiley (1984), to describe a severely mentally handicapped patient demonstrates the substantial risk of denial of human dignity that these people faced from their professional carers.

the existence of the most severely mentally handicapped patient is merely vegetative. The patient is mute, completely helpless and lies in his cot showing no awareness of his surroundings, doubly incontinent, and throughout his life requires the same nursing attention as a small baby. (Heaton-Ward and Wiley 1984: 68)

This also demonstrates the dominance of the medical model, in institutional care (for a definition of the medical model see Chapter 2) which meant that people were given a negative prognosis and were perceived according to their conditions and deficits (Boxall 2002); this resulted in negative attitudes and low expectations. Today there remains ignorance in the general public, and professionals about people with profound intellectual disabilities and their complex needs (Gates 2007). A recent study by Lewis and Stenfert-Kroese (2009) of general nursing staff attitudes towards patients with an intellectual disability found that staff reported less positive attitudes towards patients with intellectual disability than to others. They suggest that there is a risk that the lack of positive attitudes will potentially affect the quality of care given. Furthermore, according to Gates (2007) it is not unusual for people to report never seeing or meeting a person with PIMD; one explanation for this offered by Gates is the effect of institutionalisation where people were shut away from society. Their noticeable absence may also be due to the relatively few numbers of people with PIMD in the general population – currently approximately 16,000 people in England (Emerson 2009).

Mansell (2010) suggests that the relatively small number of affected people should make it easier for services to improve. However, even in the second decade of the twenty-first century following the widespread closure of long-stay institutional provision people with intellectual disability remain one of the most socially excluded groups in society (Bollard 2009). Although much progress has been made with services more focused on 'partnership and empowerment' where person-centred care is fundamental to this way of working (Jukes and Aldridge 2007), it remains of great concern that examples of abusive and discriminatory service provision still occur (Commission for Healthcare Audit and Inspection 2006, 2007; Mencap 2010). Goble (2008) discusses the notion of 'institutional abuse', explaining that disabled people have the right to experience the same quality of life as non-disabled citizens, and violation of this right is akin to institutional racism or sexism.

Risks for people with PIMD

People with PIMD are an exceptionally vulnerable group in society, and in the following section the factors contributing to this vulnerability are considered.

The need to reduce social exclusion of people with intellectual disabilities has been a matter of concern in the UK for some years, and to some extent has been addressed in both *Valuing People* (Department of Health 2001) and *Valuing People Now* (Department of Health 2009). Despite good intentions, however, it would appear that the impact of the more recent publication on the inclusion of people with PIMD is likely to be minimal without additional political commitment (Dawkins 2009). Rooney (2002) pronounced the social inclusion of PIMD as a 'myth', noting that the 'deprivation of contact and supportive networks' frequently experienced in their lives constituted 'psychological abuse' (Department of Health 2000: 9). The Department of Health also includes in its definition of psychological abuse 'emotional abuse, threats of harm or abandonment ... humiliation ... controlling ... verbal abuse ... [and] isolation ... from services'. Given the social neglect experienced by people with PIMD and their families, it is possible to claim that psychological abuse of these individuals (and often their carers) is widespread in the UK. Society's labelling of the unfortunate members of this group as 'not fully human' (Mansell 2010) seems particularly poignant in this regard.

CASE STUDY

Maureen is 38 years old, and has PIMD. As a young teenager, she was admitted to a large institution for residential care, and ten years ago moved into her present home, a shared group house a mile or two outside a busy town. Maureen's communication is at a pre-intentional level (meaning that she is unaware of the potential ability of those around her to respond), and includes a frequently repeated non-verbal moaning sound; this is rather loud. She has rarely been seen to smile, and her facial expression is characteristically immobile and unvarying in nature. Despite this, she appears to enjoy most meals and drinks, and makes no objection to being taken out in her wheelchair. Maureen's moaning increases on entering any kind of transport, and in crowded situations, but opinion is divided on whether this signifies resentment. As a result, Maureen's excursions from her home are rather limited in comparison to her peers.

CHALLENGE

■ How could those supporting Maureen help to include her more in society?

In considering your response to the above challenge, you may have considered how communication with Maureen could be made more effective – by doing so, it may become possible to ascertain some meaning in her repeated vocalisation, and therefore have a more accurate interpretation of her preferences. The team supporting her would undoubtedly need the guidance of a speech and language therapist in this attempt, who may recommend the deployment of specialist communication techniques such as intensive interaction (see below), or less formal measures such as the use of detailed observation and recording of Maureen's responses to different experiences. If it is decided that Maureen is indeed registering her objections to travel in the restricted space of any kind of motor vehicle, then efforts might be made to help her get used to this experience – or, should these prove unsuccessful, then alternative means of access to community resources (perhaps solitary use of a high-roofed minibus?) explored. Maureen would then be able to explore new experiences available in the locality – and perhaps some further afield – thus assisting her greater inclusion in the community.

The extent of the individual's care needs may also result in them being in the care and the responsibility of many agencies. It has been noted that simply being in receipt of care enhances the risks to personal safety, through 'institutional abuse' (Department of Health 2000). The Healthcare Commission has reported on the ill treatment of learning disabled service users in Cornwall (Commission for Healthcare Audit and Inspection 2006) and Sutton and Merton (Commission for Healthcare Audit and Inspection 2007). Both reports gave disturbing accounts of abuses that included dehumanising treatments, widespread lack of meaningful activity for the clients, inexpert care practices, lack of personalisation, inappropriate restraint, and physical and sexual abuse. In each case, the authors attribute these practices to a lack of staff training, poor management, inadequate resources and poor commissioning of services. The report into the Sutton and Merton service also identified institutionalised service users as being at risk from their peers, in an environment where staff were poorly versed in the procedures relating to the protection of vulnerable adults. In response to both investigations, the Healthcare Commission published a national audit of in-patient health services for people with a learning disability (Healthcare Commission 2007), recommending a wide range of measures to be taken by local and national commissioners and providers to offer an improved service, with fewer risks, to such vulnerable clients. The risks to Maureen and others may be fewer as a result, but that cannot yet be certain, as there is no evidence to demonstrate the success of this initiative.

The audit concerned residential services provided by the NHS and private sector; however, the history of literature describing the experiences of people with learning disabilities in acute health care services also reveals widespread and well-established evidence of unmet need, and exceptionally poor outcomes (Michael 2008; Emerson and Baines 2010). The causes of poor outcomes are identified as ignorance, prejudice, inadequate communication and a lack of interest in collaboration. Some of this evidence suggests that it is people with more complex disabilities who may be at more risk from professional ignorance and discrimination (Mencap 2006b) and some indicates that it is the mere presence of profound disability that necessarily brings risks additional to those already well known and articulated for the wider client group (Mansell 2010).

The risk of sexual abuse

It has been claimed recently that all people with learning disabilities are at risk of being denied access to information concerning sexual health, and are commonly denied access to those factors in UK society which encourage or support sexual expression (Richards *et al.*, in Owen and Griffiths 2009); as a result, they are at greater risk of sexual abuse, exploitation and sexually transmitted infection (see

Androulla's case study in Chapter 4 for further exploration of rights and risks for people with a learning disability). There is a lack of literature on the sexual experiences of people with profound intellectual and multiple disabilities but in one study (Murphy *et al.* 2007) of 18 subjects with PIMD referred to psychology services as the result of abuse, 15 were alleged by their carers to have been victims of sexual abuse. Sixteen of the victims were using either respite or residential services at the time of the abuse, hence supporting evidence from the Healthcare Commission of the risk presented by the mere fact of being in receipt of services.

CHALLENGE

What do you think is meant by 'sexual abuse'? Why might people like Maureen be vulnerable?

Brown and Turk (1992) claimed that sexual abuse can be defined by an individual's inability to comprehend

- the nature of sexual activity and abuse
- the moral value of the sexual act
- the possible consequences of sexual activity
- the meaning of sexual taboos.

People with PIMD in receipt of organised care are particularly vulnerable to sexual abuse if they are unable to understand the nature of sexual activity and its consequences; females are also especially susceptible (Peckham 2007).

In view of evidence of sexual abuse in the wider learning disabled population (McCarthy and Thompson 1997; Beail and Warden 2008), the demonstration that people with PIMD are not – as once thought – at less risk due to the severity of their disabilities (O'Callaghan *et al.* 2003), and the acknowledged blurring of boundaries between the instrumental touch demanded by the physical care required by this client group and that of abusive action (Cambridge and Carnaby 2000), the possibilities of exploitation have to remain a cause for serious concern. It is helpful, however, to note that the Sexual Offences Act makes it clear that the presence of 'mental disorder' itself is sufficient to demonstrate the offences included within its provision, without the need to test the capacity of the victim to consent.

The difficulties in communication for and with an individual with PIMD have already been commented upon, and the relationship to frequent social exclusion made clear; however, consideration must also be given to further risks that may not be so explicit. One such is the potential abuse of PIMD individuals whose communication may be misinterpreted (Grove *et al.* 2001) – or even ignored. The difficulties of securing evidence from people with severe or profound disabilities who have been abused is of course an additional problem, and likely to mean that cases are unlikely to reach court and convincing evidence harder to obtain (Murphy *et al.* 2007). It is possible that when the potential autonomy of people within this client group is threatened by the failure of services to include them in person-centred planning (PMLD Network 2008), and when there is widespread misinterpretation of their communication by carers (Banat *et al.* 2002), that abuses of consent – with consequent insults to self-direction – will occur.

Positive risk taking

The white paper *Valuing People* (Department of Health 2001), makes no mention of autonomy, but included in its key principles is the value of 'independence', and allies this to the observance of legal and civil rights for people with a learning disability. This represented a significant challenge to many services, which have been described as being more inclined to over-protection than to the encouragement of real independence with the risk-taking that that concept necessarily involves (Titterton 2004). Indeed, a greater degree of intellectual disability has been found to correlate both with a lack of opportunity to exercise choice and poor quality of life (Nota *et al.* 2007), the authors in addition acknowledging the influence of such factors as environment and choice opportunity; hence, it is not so much the profundity of the disability itself that results in lack of self-direction, as the poor quality of support that affected individuals are likely to enjoy.

Although risk is often understood in social care to indicate only a potentially negative outcome, it has been noted that outside this context the possibility of *benefit* to the individual may be implicit (Alaszewski 1998), and positive risk-taking may therefore be seen as an important aspect of the quality of life of people with learning disabilities – despite 'safety' being a frequent inclusion in tools designed to measure the concept (Jenkins 2002). It is perhaps because of the prioritisation of safety over inclusion for people with PIMD that the UK government's re-enforcement of *Valuing People*, the publication *Valuing People Now* (Department of Health 2009) acknowledged that they had been largely left out of the action initiated by the White Paper. However, the Healthcare Commission report *A Life Like No Other* (2007) makes clear the centrality of effective risk management to person-centred care, and the link between risk, social inclusion and responsibility has been made clear by at least one highly respected author on learning disability (Gates 2007: 182).

CASE STUDY

Ben is 26 years old, and has PIMD. He is fully mobile and very energetic; some people describe him as 'hyperactive'. He has been diagnosed with autistic spectrum disorder, and one of the ways in which this manifests itself is an apparently obsessive fascination with moving water and the patterns it makes. Hence, in the group home that he

➔

➡️

shares with five other people, Ben repeatedly runs into the bathroom to flush the toilet, an action that seems to thrill him immensely. If escorted out for a walk – an activity he seems to enjoy very much, especially if the route passes a fast moving stream or railway line (trains are another one of his favourite interests) – he compensates for the absence of water closets by repeatedly spitting on himself and playing with the saliva, or by spitting at others if they unwittingly enter his preferred and unusually large personal space. There are therefore many concerns amongst his carers about infection control, Ben's dignity and relationships with members of the local community.

CHALLENGE

■ How can this risk be managed in order to maximise Ben's social inclusion?

In developing your answer to the challenge posed, you may have identified the need to reduce the incidence of Ben's spitting behaviour as a necessary precursor to his greater social inclusion. Such an attempt would necessitate close collaboration between Ben's carers and a clinical psychologist – but would have to precede any attempt to integrate Ben more effectively into his local community.

Approaches that promote the rights of people with PIMD

The promotion of social inclusion for people with PIMD necessitates the management of risk. Many models of risk management include consideration of the capacity of the individual to learn in order to minimise the danger of harm, for example the 'competence to learn' element identified by Beck, Emery and Greenberg (1985, cited in Gates 2007). This may be problematic for people with PIMD, as their capacity to learn – whilst undeniably present in every individual – may not extend to the requirements of this task (PMLD Network, no date), and therefore impact upon the responsibility that is assumed in the management of risk. Hence there is a need for this responsibility to be shifted to those considering their 'best interests' (The Department of Constitutional Affairs 2007). Overriding the need for risk management is the need to ensure that the rights of the individual are fully respected. As indicated above, this has not always been the case in the past, or even currently (Healthcare Commission 2007; Joint Committee of the House of Lords and House of Commons 2009; Mansell 2010). Largely, it appears that the social exclusion of people with PIMD is a consequence of risk management; consideration of the ways in which such individuals can be included in society is therefore appropriate.

The focus of the report *Raising our Sights* (Mansell 2010) on the need to promote more effectively the social inclusion of people with PIMD also directed attention to the ways in which services could improve their provision to meet their needs (and those of their families). In a discussion of the components of good services, Mansell identified that person-centred services are the most effective; this necessitates the careful use of individual budgets, and a commitment to working across health and social care boundaries. He also identifies the need for families to be treated by services as the expert, for the promotion of advocacy for people with PIMD, and for improved demographic information about the client group to be gathered by local authorities and health services.

It has been claimed that one of the chief causes of discrimination against profoundly disabled individuals is the inability of others to decipher their non-verbal communication (Rooney 2002), and this deficiency is not restricted to the general public (Mansell 2010). Bunning (in Pawlyn and Carnaby 2009) demonstrated the application of the ecological model of communication to this client group, emphasising the environment in which communication takes place, rather than individual skills, identifying that communication partners need to take responsibility for the initiation, maintenance and development of meaningful exchange with people with PIMD. People with PIMD have the right to be informed about the actions which have an impact on their lives and also where possible have a role in decision making. Therefore how practitioners communicate is very important, those interacting with the person are recommended to develop their skills in order to promote a socially responsive environment in which the understanding of cause and effect may be fostered, and to draw upon such supports as multisensory environments, multimedia techniques and objects of reference in order to boost the effectiveness of their communication. Bunning also emphasises the need for all those in the social vicinity of the person to negotiate and review regularly their observations and techniques with the individual for the purpose of ensuring the usefulness of their approach.

Some systems of communication with people with PIMD have proved sufficiently successful to have been 'branded'. One such is *intensive interaction*, developed initially by Ephraim and later advanced by Nind and Hewett (2001). Intensive interaction is an approach that seeks to foster a greater sense of empathy between a person with autism and/or profound learning disabilities and a supporter, laying emphasis upon the need for the latter to make a conscious effort to enter the other person's inner world. This effort might be communicated by the supporter imitating stereotypical behaviours (e.g. hand-flapping, or string-flicking), engaging responsive eye contact, echoing vocalisations and/or taking up a position of close physical proximity with the aim of demonstrating rapport with their communication partner (Firth 2008). Intensive interaction may be engaged simply as an activity of value in its own right, or as one with a developmental target for the client, but its potential for promoting greater social inclusion is clear (Firth 2008).

Person Centred Active Support (PCAS) is a technique, developed principally for people with profound disabilities, that seeks to engage the individual in activity that is meaningful for them and which promotes their inclusion in 'everyday' life (Person Centred Active Support 2010). As often the case with intensive interaction, the aim is not necessarily a developmental one, but one based on the primacy of self-direction, and the notion that by taking part in their chosen activities, people will be able to improve the quality of their lives. The chief constituents of PCAS are a communication strategy designed to meet the needs and preferences of the individual, combined with elements of positive behavioural support (Ashman and Beadle-Brown 2006). Research has demonstrated the efficacy of the approach, which requires significant commitment from organisations and staff at all levels if it is to succeed (Beadle-Brown *et al.* 2008).

Another source of useful guidance when communicating with people with PIMD are the *See What I Mean* (SWIM) *Guidelines*, developed by Grove *et al.* (2000). Their primary intention is to provide an aid to decision making, but through their acknowledgement of the ambiguities and ambivalence inherent in any human communication, they can also encourage those interacting with clients to exchange interpretations of behaviours and conduct comparative exercises in order to establish probable meanings. Hence although their principal use may be in assisting the individual to participate in major decisions (e.g. during transition, or regarding the expenditure of a personal budget), they have the potential to improve the quality of the immediate communication environment.

Good services focus on quality of staff relationships with the disabled person (Mansell 2010), and whilst health and social care professionals can – and should – engage with the initiatives of national government and local agencies to promote the rights of people with PIMD, a good place to start for the individual practitioner is with the development of his or her communication skills with this very particular client group.

Conclusion

This chapter has considered the rights, risks and – to the limited extent that is possible – responsibilities of people with profound intellectual and multiple disabilities. The 'care' to which individuals have been exposed in the past, and those to which they may be subject today, have been discussed, with an invitation to the reader to reflect upon the resultant social exclusion of this group of people. Case studies have been presented to offer an opportunity to develop thinking about the needs of people with PIMD, with particular regard to social inclusion and communication, and information concerning potentially useful communication strategies presented. It is hoped that the reader will be equipped, at the conclusion of this chapter, with the awareness and knowledge required in order to develop their skills and promote the inclusion and safety of some of the most vulnerable members of society.

References

Alaszewski, A. (1998) *Risk, Health and Welfare: Policies, Strategies and Practice.* Buckingham: Open University Press.

Allen, P. (2009) Mental deficiency institutions: have the obituaries been fair and balanced? In M. Jukes (ed.), *Learning Disability Nursing Practice.* London: Quay Books.

APA (American Psychiatric Association) (2000) *Diagnostic and Statistical Manual of Mental Disorders, 4th edition: Text Revision.* Washington DC: APA.

Arbus, D. (1995) *Untitled.* New York: Aperture.

Ashman, B. and Beadle-Brown, J. (2006) *A Valued Life: Developing Person-centred Approaches so that People Can Be More Included.* London: United Response.

Banat, D., Summers, S. and Pring, T. (2002) An investigation into carers' perceptions of the verbal comprehension ability of adults with severe learning disabilities. *British Journal of Learning Disabilities,* 30(2): 78–81.

Beadle-Brown, J., Hutchinson, A. and Whelton, B. (2008) A better life: the implementation and effect of person centred active support in The Avenues Trust. *Tizard Learning Disability Review,* 13(4): 15–24.

Beail, N. and Warden, S. (2008) Sexual abuse of adults with learning disabilities. *Journal of Intellectual Disability Research,* 39(5): 382–7.

Beck, A. T., Emery, G. and Greenberg, T. (1985) *Anxiety Disorders and Phobias: A Cognitive Perspective.* New York: Basic Books.

Blatt, B. and Kaplan, F. (1974) *Christmas in Purgatory: A Photographic Essay on Mental Retardation.* Second Syracuse, NY: Human Policy Press.

Bogdan, R. and Taylor, S. (1994) *The Social Meaning of Mental Retardation Two Life Stories.* London: Teachers College Press.

Bollard, M. (ed.) (2009) *Intellectual Disability and Social Inclusion: A Critical Review.* London: Churchill Livingstone Elsevier.

Boxall, K. (2002) Individual and social models of disability and the experiences of people with learning difficulties. In D. Race (ed.), *Learning Disability: A Social Approach.* London: Routledge.

Brown, H. and Turk, V. (1992) Defining sexual abuse as it affects adults with learning disabilities. *Mental Handicap,* 20: 44–55.

Cambridge, P. and Carnaby, S. (2000) A personal touch: managing the risks of abuse during intimate and personal care. *Journal of Adult Protection,* 2: 4–16.

Commission for Healthcare Audit and Inspection (2006) Joint investigation into the provision of services for people with learning disabilities at Cornwall Partnership NHS Trust. London: CHAI (online). Available at: http://www.cqc.org.uk/_db/_documents/cornwall_investigation_report.pdf (accessed 25 May 2010).

Commission for Healthcare Audit and Inspection (2007) Investigation into the service for people with learning disabilities provided by Sutton and Merton Primary Care Trust. London: CHAI (online). Available at: http://www.cqc.org.uk/_db/_documents/Sutton_and_Merton_inv_Main_Tag.pdf (accessed 25 May 2010).

Dawkins, B. (2009) Valuing Tom: will *Valuing People Now* change the lives of people with profound and multiple learning disabilities? *Tizard Learning Disability Review,* 14(4): 3–11.

Deacon, J. (1974) *Tongue Tied: Fifty Years of Friendship in a Subnormality Hospital.* Available at: http://tonguetied.hostoi.com/ (accessed 29 December 2010).

The Department of Constitutional Affairs (2007) *MCA Code of Practice.* London: TSO.

Department of Health (2000) *No Secrets: Guidance on Developing and Implementing Multi-agency Policies and Procedures to Protect Vulnerable Adults from Abuse.* London: Department of Health.

Department of Health (2001) *Valuing People: A New Strategy for Learning Disability for the 21st Century*. London: Department of Health.

Department of Health (2003) *Sexual Offences Act 2003*. Available at http://www.statutelaw.gov.uk/content.aspx?activeTextDocId=820904 (accessed 5 November 2010).

Department of Health (2008) *Healthcare for All: Report of the independent Inquiry into Access to Healthcare for People with Learning Disabilities*. London: Department of Health.

Department of Health (2009) *Valuing People Now: A New Three-year Strategy for People with Learning Disabilities*. London: Department of Health.

Ellis, D. (1982) Joey Deacon: a suitable case for labelling? *Developmental Medicine Child Neurology*, 24(4): 485–8.

Emerson, E. (2009) Estimating future numbers of adults with profound multiple learning disabilities in England. *Tizard Learning Disability Review*, 14(4): 49–55.

Emerson, E. and Baines, S. (2010) *Health Inequalities and People with Learning Disabilities in the UK: 2010*. Improving Health and Lives: Learning Disability Observatory.

Firth, G. (2008) A dual aspect process model of intensive interaction. *British Journal of Learning Disabilities*, 37: 43–9.

Gates, B. (ed.) (2007) *Learning Disabilities: Toward Inclusion* (5th edn). London: Churchill Livingstone.

Goble, C. (2008) Institutional abuse. In J. Swain and S. French (eds), *Disability on Equal Terms*. London: Sage Publications.

Grove, N., Bunning, K., Porter, J. and Morgan, M. (2000) *See What I Mean: Guidelines to Aid Understanding of Communication by People with Severe and Profound Learning Disabilities*. Kidderminster: BILD and Mencap.

Grove, N., Bunning, K. and Porter, J. (2001) Interpreting the meaning of behaviour by people with intellectual disabilities: theoretical and methodological issues. In F. Columbus (ed.), *Advances in Psychology Research*, Vol. 7. New York: Nova Science.

Healthcare Commission (2007) *A Life Like No Other: A National Audit of Specialist Inpatient Healthcare Services for People with Learning Difficulties in England*. London: Healthcare Commission.

Heaton-Ward, A. (1978) *Left Behind: Study of Mental Handicap* (Psychiatric topics for community workers). London: Routledge.

Heaton-Ward, A. and Wiley, Y. (1984) *Mental Handicap* (5th edn). Bristol: Wright.

IASSID (no date) *Profound Multiple Disabilities Mission*. Available at: http://www.iassid.org/sirgs/profound-multiple-disabilities (accessed 29 December 2010).

ITN (1981) *News at Ten: 'Silent Minority'*. United Kingdom: NFO Newsfilm Online.

Jenkins, R. (2002) Enhancing quality of life for people with learning disabilities. *Learning Disability Practice*, 5(9): 29–35.

Joint Committee of the House of Lords and House of Commons on Human Rights (2009) *A Life Like Any Other? Human Rights of Adults with Learning Disabilities*. London: The Stationery Office.

Jukes, M. and Aldridge, J. (eds) (2007) *Person-centred Practices: A Holistic and Integrated Approach*. London: Quay Books.

Lewis, S. and Stenfert-Kroese, B. (2009) An investigation of nursing staff attitudes and emotional reactions towards patients with intellectual disability in a general hospital setting. *Journal of Applied Research in Intellectual Disabilities*, 23(4): 355–65.

Mansell, J. (2010) *Raising our Sights: Services for Adults with Profound Intellectual and Multiple Disabilities*. Canterbury: Tizard Centre, University of Kent.

McCarthy, M. and Thompson, D. (1997) A prevalence study of sexual abuse of adults with intellectual disabilities referred for sex education. *Journal of Applied Research in Learning Disabilities*, 10(2): 105–24.

McClimens, A. and Richardson, M. (2010) Social constructions and social models: disability explained? In G. Grant, P. Ramcharan, M. Flynn and M. Richardson (eds), *Learning Disability: A Lifecycle Approach*. Maidenhead: McGraw-Hill.

Mencap (2001) *No Ordinary Life: The Support Needs of Families Caring for Children and Adults with Profound and Multiple Learning Disabilities*. London: Royal Society for Mentally Handicapped Children and Adults.

Mencap (2006a) *Meet the People*, CD-ROM. London: Mencap.

Mencap (2006b) *Breaking Point – Families Still Need a Break: A Report on the Continuing Problem of Caring Without a Break for Children and Adults with Severe and Profound Learning Disabilities*. London: Mencap.

Mencap (2010) *Communication and People with the Most Complex Needs: What Works and Why This is Essential*. London: Mencap.

Michael, J. (2008) *Healthcare for All: Report of the Independent Inquiry into Access to Healthcare for People with Learning Disabilities*. London: Department of Health.

Morris, P. (1969) *Put Away: A Sociological Study of Institutions for the Mentally Retarded*. London: Routledge & Kegan Paul.

Murphy, G., O'Callaghan, A. C. and Clare, I. C. H. (2007) The impact of alleged abuse on behaviour in adults with severe intellectual disabilities. *Journal of Intellectual Disability Research*, 51(10): 741–9.

Nind, M. and Hewett, D. (2001) *A Practical Guide to Intensive Interaction*. Kidderminster: British Institute for Learning Disability.

Nota, L., Ferrari, L., Soresi, S. and Wehmeyer, M. (2007) Self-determination, social abilities and the quality of life of people with intellectual disability. *Journal of Intellectual Disability Research*, 51(11): 850–65.

O'Callaghan, A., Murphy, G. and Clare, I. (2003) The impact of abuse on men and women with severe learning disabilities and their families. *British Journal of Learning Disabilities*, 31: 175–80.

Owen, F. and Griffiths, D. (2009) *Challenges to the Human Rights of People with Intellectual Disabilities*. London: Jessica Kingsley.

Pawlyn, J. and Carnaby, S. (2009) *Profound Intellectual and Multiple Disabilities: Nursing Complex Needs*. Chichester: Wiley Blackwell.

Peckham, N. (2007) The vulnerability and sexual abuse of people with learning disabilities. *British Journal of Learning Disabilities*, 35: 131–7.

Person Centred Active Support (2010) What is person-centred active support? Available at: http://www.personcentredactivesupport.com/aboutperson-centredactivesupport (accessed 27 September 2010).

PMLD Network (no date) About profound and multiple learning disabilities. Available at: http://www.pmldnetwork.org/ (accessed 27 September 2010).

PMLD Network (2008) PMLD Network response to *Valuing People Now*. Available at http://www.pmldnetwork.org/what_do_we_want/valuing_people_now-pmld_network_response.doc (accessed 27 September 2010).

Race, D. (ed.) (2002) *Learning Disability: A Social Approach*. London: Routledge.

Rooney, S. (2002) Social inclusion and people with profound and multiple disabilities: reality or myth? In D. Race (ed.), *Learning Disability: A Social Approach*. London: Routledge.

Ryan, J. and Thomas, F. (1987) *The Politics of Mental Handicap Revised Edition*. London: Free Association Books.

Silent Minority (1981) Directed by Nigel Evans (Video cassette). Great Britain: ATV.

Titterton, M. (2004) *Risk and Risk-Taking in Health and Social Welfare*. London: Jessica Kingsley.

World Health Organisation (1993) *International Classification of Diseases 10th edition: Diagnostic Criteria for Research*. Geneva: World Health Organisation.

Risk, Informed Practice and the Non-specialist Practitioner: Towards More Effective Work with Those Who Misuse Substances

Bob Cecil

Introduction

This chapter is written for non-specialist health and social care practitioners whose work brings them into contact with people who misuse substances. Central to the discussion is consideration of how practitioners conceptualize and work with risk in a complex and changing practice and policy landscape. In keeping with the other contributors to this book, the three Rs – rights, risks and responsibilities – form the framework for discussion. To focus the attention of the reader on the most salient elements of a very wide area of study, the chapter is separated into three main sections.

First, the chapter introduces the key concepts and intervention approaches followed by an exploration of the wider context and definitions of 'risk' within health and social care, including social work.

The next part of the chapter aims to help practitioners develop a more informed approach to their assessment of risk and decision making, emphasising those factors which can enhance or obstruct a fair, accountable, informed and objective approach to working with substance misusers.

Finally, the chapter addresses frameworks for practice and assessment. It aims to show how the key ingredients of the non-specialist's training – the knowledge, skills and values that are needed to help people address a range of other life problems – may be applied to help practitioners work effectively with people who misuse substances.

Throughout the chapter practice-based vignettes and examples are used to illustrate particular discussion points, and exercises and questions are included to help maximise and enhance learning.

LEARNING OUTCOMES

By the end of the chapter you should have developed your understanding of:

- The definition, scope and social construction of substance misuse

- Key ethical and treatment debates and discourses and different treatment approaches to dealing with problem drinking and the misuse of drugs and other substances

- The application of theories and models of risk assessment to different scenarios involving values-based and ethical challenges

- The importance of inter-professional and collaborative working in managing complexity whilst recognising the limits of personal and professional responsibilities.

Discussion throughout the chapter will address a number of questions including the following:

- What constitutes informed and competent practice on the part of practitioners in relation to the (risk) assessment and management of drug and alcohol related problems?

- What does an informed choice in relation to drug and alcohol use look like on the part of service users?

- To what extent should practitioners be responsible for adopting an educative stance in their work with this service user group?

- How do we ensure that the right of service users and carers to an effective, knowledge-based, non-stigmatising and evidence-informed service is addressed?

- How do we accommodate/reconcile respect for the right to make a lifestyle choice/service user self-determination in the light of harmful and damaging behaviour?

As it is beyond the scope of the chapter to provide a definitive guide to substance misuse, the reader is signposted to relevant sources at the end of the chapter.

Understanding substance misuse, social constructionism and the importance of definition

There are many explanations as to why people may develop problems with drugs, alcohol and other substances. Similarly, there is no single, definitive definition of a 'substance'. Many books on the subject (e.g. Pycroft 2010; Allan 2010; Shephard 1990) start by considering the terminology used within the substance misuse field and go on to look at the range of definitions available. Such a definition is important for several reasons; the process of defining helps put a boundary around a particular topic to help conceptualise the subject, and identify the scope of related issues. The language used is also significant; it conveys meaning and indicates ways in which phenomena and social problems may be perceived.

CHALLENGE

List all the words and terms that you have heard to describe people who use alcohol and other drugs.

■ Are they positive or negative?

■ What image comes to mind in relation to each word listed?

■ Do your answers show that you think the person who uses substances *is* a problem or *has* a problem?

In addition to defining substance misuse we can also consider how it is socially constructed as a problem. Social constructionism (Burr 1996) is a theory which is interested in exploring the ways in which individuals and groups construct their perception of the world. It is interested in how those phenomena come to be socially constructed and defined. Meaning and power are both concepts central to the theory. How 'substance misuse' is constructed – in the same way as 'adolescence', 'old age' or 'risk' comes to be constructed – will have implications for how practitioners view 'the substance misuser' or the behaviour/issues associated with substance misuse.

> Each society has its own culturally and socially sanctioned explanation ... for phenomena such as illness, poverty, failure, success, violence, crime. (Augoustinos 1998: 62)

Part of professional and responsible practice should involve practitioners questioning how they have come to hold particular beliefs. Macdonald and Patterson (1991: 19) provide a useful introduction to guide this reflective process by identifying three key components of attitudes:

1. They are *descriptive* – 'Drug users look dirty ...'

2. They are *evaluative* – 'Drug users are sick/bad people.'

3. They are *prescriptive* – 'Drug users should be given long prison sentences.'

By practitioners confronting and then understanding why they hold particular stereotypes, biased opinions and assumptions, it may facilitate a more objective understanding of those who use substances. Macdonald and Patterson (1991: 22–3) also offer a framework to help practitioners understand how they conceptualise drug use. They identify four positions:

1. *Moral:* Where the drug user is seen as a 'weak' person who may even be acting in a 'depraved' or 'evil' manner.

2. *Medical:* Where the drug user is seen as 'sick' or 'ill' person that therefore needs medical treatment.

3. *Legal:* Where the drug user is seen as a 'bad' or 'wicked' person who engages in rational criminal activity. Punishment is seen as the solution.

4. *Social and political:* Here there are several perceptions of substance misusers. For example, as a 'normal' person whose drug use has developed as a strategy for coping with life's strains and pressures. Alternatively, as a 'victim' of a particular social environment characterised by high degrees of social, economic or emotional deprivation or finally the notion of the 'normalisation' applies where substance use is seen as an enjoyable, recreational human activity within certain social groups.

Language is an important part of this process as it is through language that 'our shared versions of knowledge are constructed' (Burr 1996: 2). For example in the UK drug users who have stopped using drugs are often referred to as being 'clean'. Does this mean that the individual still currently using drugs is therefore 'dirty'? Clearly the attitudes, labels and the views held by practitioners will be central to how they engage and work with substance misusers, and also affect how the practitioner understands and frames the concept of 'problem substance misuse'. The substance misuser who refuses to accept/refutes the label of 'addict' or 'alcoholic' may indeed *not* be 'in denial'. They may be perfectly happy to speak in detail about their use of a particular substance or underlying problems but simply choose not to associate themselves with the label of 'alcoholic' or 'addict' if for the individual concerned, that label has a negative connotation or image. Conversely, for the individuals who now choose to define themselves as 'an alcoholic' or 'addict', it may represent a cognitive shift in how they view themselves and realisation that they do have a problem with a particular substance.

In the same way as how a substance is defined, and the language used is important, so too, is how 'substance misuse' is defined. As a reference point for this chapter, the following Advisory Council on the Misuse of Drugs (ACMD 2006) definition will be used:

■ The term 'drugs' refers to all psychoactive substances which are used to alter thoughts, feelings and actions. These include those which can be legally sold, purchased or possessed (albeit often with restrictions), and those which are illegal under the Misuse of Drugs Act (1971) in the UK or the equivalent legislation on other jurisdictions

- Drug use or substance use is drug taking for example in the form of inges-tion through smoking, drinking or swallowing or through injecting
- Drug use or substance use is drug taking judged to be inappropriate or dangerous
- Drug addiction or dependence is characterized by strong compulsions to take a drug/s and difficulty in stopping despite harmful consequences. (ACMD 2006: 15)

In keeping with other literature from the field (Allan 2010: 142), the generic term 'substance' will be used in this chapter unless direct reference to a partic-ular drug is needed.

Substance misuse: nature and scope

Reflecting the multi-faceted nature and impact of drug use, the ACMD also defines the problem drug user as 'anyone who experiences social, physical, legal or psychological problems with one or more drugs' (ACMD 2006: 15).This definition is important as it introduces the concept of 'problem substance misuse' acknowledging the breadth of areas which can potentially be effected by substance misuse and moves away from a very narrow definition which the terms 'alcoholic' or 'addict ' can imply (Miller and Rollnick 1991). Increasingly the term 'problem substance misusers' is used 'to refer to those whose use of alcohol or other drugs causes financial, legal, social, psychological and/or health problems for themselves *or for others*' (McKellar and Coggans 1997: 53, author's italics) and as such encompasses the wide range of problems that may result from the use of substances in society.

As Pycroft (2010: 4) observes, there is a 'nexus of problems that can become involved with the use of substances even legal ones'. He continues that these may be either bio-psychological in nature (for example, severe withdrawal symptoms from alcohol or heroin) or socially constructed (for example, making the use of certain drugs a criminal offence). However, 'Our starting point should not be legality, or the contemporaneous status quo, but the evidence available for the nature of particular drugs and the nature of their benefits and harms. This has to involve a hard-nosed and realistic comparison of the nature of risk for each substance' (Pycroft 2010: 4).

It is useful to group substances into the following six categories, based on Pycroft (2010) and Edwards (2004):

1. Sedatives: Substances which slow the functioning of the brain and include alcohol, benzodiazepines and barbiturates.

2. Stimulants: Drugs like amphetamines and cocaine which lead to increased heart rate, agitation/excitability and can lead to paranoia.

3. Opiates: Drugs which reduce pain and include opiate narcotics such as opium, heroin, methadone.

4. Hallucinogens: Drugs that alter perception such as Datura (magic mushrooms), Lysergic Acid Diethylamide (LSD).

5. Mixed effects: Drugs such as Ecstasy which alter perception, stimulate and may lead to hallucinations.

6. Volatiles: Including solvents which can lead to euphoria and excitement and depressed reflexes.

Dependence on substances can take two forms:

1. Physical dependence is a state which occurs only with certain classes of drug such as opiates, alcohol, barbiturates and minor tranquillisers. Tolerance refers to the way in which the body adjusts its functioning as it becomes accustomed to the drug's presence. Larger doses are then needed to achieve the same effects. If the drug is suddenly removed, the body can go into a state of withdrawal. The type and severity of the withdrawal is also determined to a large extent by psychological and situational factors.

2. Psychological dependence can be said to exist when a person has a strong desire or craving to continue taking a drug and it has become difficult or seemingly impossible to stop despite adverse and harmful consequences.

Risk and vulnerability: exploring the context and key debates

Returning to the scope of 'problem substance use', consider the National Treatment Outcome Research study (NTORS) (Gossop *et al.* 2003), which revealed that the partners of 38 per cent of those seeking treatment also used drugs and female substance misusers were more likely to have a drug-using partner. Around half of those seeking treatment had children younger than 16 years of age (cited in Pycroft 2010: 18). Such studies provide vital information in relation to the profile of those using substances as well as the scope and nature of substance misuse itself.

They also provide important data for the conscientious practitioner and a framework within which other research findings can be located. For example, taking family systems and context, Forrester and Harwin (2006) examined the effects of parental substance misuse (PSM) within child care social work. They found that substance misuse featured in 34 per cent of the 290 cases studied and that families involving substance misuse were more vulnerable on a variety of measures: the children were younger, the parents had more individual problems and the families lived in more difficult social situations (Forrester and Harwin 2006: 325).

Such findings have led some to propose a social model of risk (Parsloe 1999) which acknowledges the importance and dynamic interplay of environmental factors such as poverty, poor housing and ill health as well as the quality of social networks as central to good practice. Through the reconstruction of substance misusers as 'vulnerable' as opposed to 'dangerous' and viewing them in the context of their wider life experience, we begin to see that working with substance misusers does not require the practitioner to have an intimate knowledge of all substances, but rather what is needed is a clear perception on the practitioner's part of the problems and issues that face substance misusers (Goodman 2007: 8).

The two real-life studies below can help you to become more aware of your own attitudes towards people who misuse substances. Answer the following questions as honestly as you can; this will also help you think about your own role as a practitioner in such situations.

CASE STUDY

Consider the following, which was the subject of a serious case review in Manchester in 2010 where Tracy Sutherland, a mother with a history of heavy alcohol use, was jailed for 27 months for neglect, following the death of her 13-month-old son, Alexander (known in the serious case review report as 'Child T'). The report stated that his mother 'experienced abuse as a child and seriously abused alcohol, which led to neglect and weight loss. Despite failed multi-agency attempts to work with the mother, and repeated referrals from relatives, Child T remained in her care. Child T died strapped into his buggy in front of a gas fire. He had been dead for a number of days when discovered. The review identifies similarities to other child deaths in Manchester; including a failure to assess the impact alcohol has on parenting capacity, and failing to focus on the child' (Muir 2011).

Similarly Ofsted's evaluation of serious case reviews from 1 April 2009 to 31 March 2010 cites a further case about 'two boys whose mother acknowledged that she had a problem relating to misuse of alcohol. However, this was not assessed to see whether it was a significant issue. The link was not made between her alcohol misuse and her capacity to act as a parent to the children. The review found that agencies involved had not taken sufficient notice of the father's concerns about his partner's drinking' (Ofsted 2010).

CHALLENGE

■ What is your initial response to each of these situations?

■ Why do you think the agencies failed to recognise the risks these children were exposed to?

■ How could staff be trained to be more challenging and assertive when working with parents who misuse substances in order to avoid tragic consequences such as the death of a child?

■ What are your thoughts about balancing the rights of parents who may misuse substances and the rights of their children? Where are the points of tension?

These are complex questions which have been explored in recent reviews of how children such as Alexander are protected. Early identification and provision of help is in the child's best interests and multi-agency services which deliver support for families are vital in promoting children's well-being (Munro 2011: 10). The Coalition Programme for Government has recently made a commitment to investigate a new approach to supporting those families with multiple problems including poor mental health, alcohol and substance misuse. A small number of exemplar areas are being used as pilots building on family interventions which adopt a multi-agency approach with an 'intensive' and 'persistent' style of working to challenge and support families. Such approaches include the Family Nurse Partnership which is a preventive programme for vulnerable first-time mothers. A second part of the strategy highlights the role of 'mentor' areas with a track record of successfully supporting families in acting as dissemination hubs to share their practice know-how (Munro 2011: 30).

In addressing the above questions and the last question in particular, perhaps you began to think about competing rights and some of the complexities involved in trying to predict harmful outcomes. In a review of relevant literature (Mitchell and Glendinning 2008: 20), three key areas of potential conflict were reported which can be played out in the following scenarios:

■ Right of service users to take risks or make the choice to undertake 'risky' behaviour and learn from experience versus the responsibility of practitioners (or others with a 'duty of care') to protect users from harm potential danger.

■ Right of service users to take risk versus the responsibility of practitioners to protect others, including members of the wider community from harm.

■ Right of service users to take risks in their own home (or other informal settings) versus the right of paid carers to have a safe working environment.

Risk taking is also based on the view of the service user as an 'active citizen' with rights and responsibilities rather than the professional as the expert (Gurney 2000). As one service user commented in research carried out by Joseph Rowntree Foundation (JRF) into drug users' involvement in decision making about treatment:

They [staff] should have an input because the doctors know what they're talking about. And I should have an input cos I know what's best for me. (Community client, England, first interview, Fischer *et al.* 2007: 12)

In a person-centred vein, Tindall (1997) also views risk taking as central to the empowerment of the individual which facilitates personal development with others highlighting an increasing emphasis on each individual's responsibility to assess and manage risk in their own life (Lupton 1999).

Theorising substance misuse: approaches to treatment and intervention

Theoretical frameworks are important in making connections and promoting practitioner knowledge of the various methods and approaches that may prove effective in relation to working with people who misuse substances, but literature can offer an additional dimension that enhances empathy and understanding by providing access to the inner life of people who use services.

In the following account the French writer Marguerite Duras describes her lifelong relationship with alcohol:

> I started drinking at parties and political meetings – glasses of wine first, then whisky. And then, when I was forty-one I met someone who really loved alcohol and drank every day, though sensibly. I soon outstripped him. That went on for ten years, until I got cirrhosis of the liver and started vomiting blood. Then I gave up drinking for ten years. That was the first time. Then I started drinking again, and gave it up again, I forget why. Then I stopped smoking but I could only do that by drinking again. This is the third time I've given up ... I became an alcoholic as soon as I started to drink. I drank like one straight away, and left everyone else behind. I began by drinking in the evening, then at midday, then in the morning, and then I began to drink every two hours. I've never drugged myself in any other way. I've always known that if I took heroin it would get out of control ... When a woman drinks it's as if an animal were drinking, or a child. Alcoholism is scandalous in a woman, and a female alcoholic is rare, a serious matter ... I'm one of those alcoholics who can be set off again by drinking just one glass of wine. I don't know the medical term for it ... And after a time you have the choice – whether to keep drinking until you're senseless and lose your identity, or to go no further than the beginnings of happiness. To die so to speak, every day, or to go on living. (Duras 1990: 15–19)

======================= **CHALLENGE** =======================

■ How do you understand Duras's alcohol use and pattern of drinking?

■ What do you see as the risks?

■ In terms of their seriousness, how would you prioritise them?

There are many ways, theoretically, that Duras's situation and use of alcohol can be understood. Listed below are some of the key theoretical approaches with key concepts highlighted which are of relevance to understanding substance misuse. The list is not exhaustive. As you read them, consider which theories you are drawn to and, importantly, why?

Substance misuse as an illness

Often referred to as the 'the disease model' this approach maintains that the condition is lifelong and irreversible and affects a specific and distinct group of people. It argues that substance misusers with the illness have lost control of their substance use and that on stopping using the substance it leads to overwhelming cravings (Shephard 1990; Pycroft 2010). This perspective underpins organisations such as Alcoholics Anonymous and Narcotics Anonymous with their adherence to Twelve Steps philosophy and is reflected in the terminology 'addict' or 'alcoholic'. Abstinence is seen as the only treatment goal.

Psychological approaches

This perspective includes a range of learning theory based perspectives including social learning, behavioural and cognitive approaches. Viewing substance misuse as a functional behaviour where the user expects to gain some benefit as well as analysis of the consequences is the bedrock of a number of specific behavioural and cognitive interventions frequently used in the treatment of substance misuse (Curran and Drummond 2007). At one end of the spectrum, behavioural psychological approaches with a very narrow 'stimulus-response' explanation based solely on conditioning do not acknowledge any sense of human agency on the part of the substance misuser. As has been observed, the human being is 'more than just a ping pong ball with a memory' who approaches situations with a range of expectations, anticipation and fears (Bannister 1966, cited in Butt and Parton 2005: 796).

Allied to this is Kelly's (1955) personal construct theory with its notion of the 'person-as-scientist'. Here the individual is 'like a scientist each with their own theories, hypotheses and experiments on which their action is based. Everyone has their own construction of events and what they do makes sense to them' (Butt and Parton 2005: 794). This theory emphasises the individual's capacity to create meaning, acknowledges the power and potential of the individual to effect change (self-efficacy) and revise personal 'systems of knowing' across time.

Sociological perspectives

These may be interested in how substance use is developed as a career (Chein 1969) or from an interactionalist perspective how users come to be labelled as 'deviant' or scapegoated as 'folk devils' within a society. The 'deviant' identity may be actively sought by some substance users for whom the very act of substance misuse can represent a means of distancing themselves from non-users. The study of other economic and social factors such as poverty or the availability of specific substances also may fall under a sociological perspective.

Types of intervention

Equally important for non-specialist practitioners is the responsibility to inform themselves about the various forms of intervention that are available. The range of services available to adult substance misusers is outlined in the Models of Care Framework (MOCF) to be commissioned throughout England and operationalised locally through the work of local Drug Action Teams. The MOCF advocates a whole systems four tier approach (Pycroft 2010: 109) and the list of interventions includes: advice and information, community prescribing, harm reduction, psychological and counselling support including cognitive-behavioural approaches, relapse prevention, motivational enhancement work and family therapy, detoxification and rehabilitation aftercare (National Treatment Agency for Substance Misuse, 2006).

Gardner (2004) also provides a very useful overview of the range of treatments available within a 'tiered' approach which is common practice in a range of health settings. The degree of expert help applied is in response to varying degrees of need. She outlines the following interventions: bibliotherapy (leaflets and books giving practical self-help information), advice, brief problem solving and support, counselling, structured groups, and formal psychotherapy (psychodynamic psychotherapy, cognitive behavioural therapy, cognitive analytic therapy or systemic or family therapy (Gardner 2004: 122).

Professional responsibilities and the informed practitioner – bias, values and person-centred practice explored

Some 20 years ago, Shephard (1990) noted reluctance among non-specialists to work with substance misusers. The reasons cited included a lack of knowledge about the substance, a lack of confidence about being able to contribute to a positive outcome and insufficient priority given to the problem within the agency. Similarly, how drugs are seen has an important bearing on how drug takers are perceived.

> Negative and ill-informed beliefs about drugs can be expected to translate themselves into negative and ill-judged reactions to users. (Griffiths and Pearson 1988: 13).

More recently a study of social work students and qualified social workers (Loughran *et al.* 2010) examined why helping professionals may still be reluctant and lack confidence in addressing alcohol and other drugs (AOD) misuse problems. The study revisited and examined role theory (Shaw *et al.* 1978) with its sub-domains of role adequacy (feeling knowledgeable about one's work) and role legitimacy (believing one has the right to address certain service user issues) and role support. Using the Drug and Drug Problems Perception Questionnaire (DDUPPQ) participants were asked to rate their responses to a number of questions which included the following:

- 'I feel I know enough about the causes of drug problems to carry out my role when working with drug users' (Role adequacy)
- 'I feel I have the right to ask a patient for any information that is relevant to their drug problems' (Role legitimacy)
- 'If I felt the need I could easily find someone who would be able to help me formulate the best approach to a drug user' (Role support). (Loughran *et al.* 2010)

Central to the work of professionals and other practitioners working with problem drug users is the concept of person-centred care. Within this approach there is an important focus on starting at where the service user is, acknowledging the individuality of each person as well as each person's right to be treated equitably and with dignity (Koubel and Bungay 2009). Its importance within the field of substance misuse has been well highlighted:

> A person-centred approach that recognizes an individual's unique biography and circumstances will not only enhance the likelihood of a positive relationship between practitioner and client, but should also provide a secure basis upon which to begin to tailor services to particular needs. (Crome *et al.* 2009: 10–11)

Key, too, is the notion of self-determination which recognises that it is the problem substance user who 'should make decisions and take the necessary steps to improve the situation wherever possible' (Thompson 2000: 110). Goodman states that substance misusers need support and encouragement to gain or regain control of their lives as 'they are no more or less deserving of support because of their habit but they may require additional assessment, resources and forms of intervention as a consequence' (Goodman 2009: 6).

Human rights discourses are becomingly increasingly important within helping professions. Central to such perspectives is the notion that needs should be participatively defined (Cemlyn 2008) and that rights are implemented through meeting those needs (Ife 2001).This is in line with the exchange model of assessment which takes as its starting point that service users should be seen as the 'expert' on themselves and their situation. A collaborative approach is seen as key to the creation of an effective working relationship where the practitioner facilitates service users to tell their stories and values the use of this material in exploring their situation (Smale *et al.* 1993, 2000).

Often, however, a number of factors can prevent practitioners adhering to the principles of person-centred practice. Bias, discrimination and an unchecked subjectivity on the practitioner's part can enter the process resulting in drug users receiving a service or approach which reflects the worker's agenda or wider societal concerns rather than being sensitive to their needs. At the micro level, the interaction, dialogue, types of questions and manner in which they are asked and both practitioners' and substance misusers' prior experience of helping/being helped all need careful attention as part of the process of establishing an effective working relationship. The practitioner's formulation of risk and risk identities is also a key factor which will be further examined in the conclud-ing section (Stanford 2010).

Learning that many service users may not always be receptive to help can be a significant part of a practitioner's development (O'Connor *et al.* 2009) and calls for a careful appreciation of the differences between the 'voluntary' and 'involuntary' service user.

Evidence also suggests that there are a number of threats to achieving effec-tive working relationships with parents who misuse drugs. For example, Forrester *et al.*'s research (2008) explores how child and family social workers talk to parents about child welfare concerns. The authors reported that 'the most striking finding was the high level of confrontation and the low level of listening shown by social workers' (Forrester *et al.* 2008: 32). The findings showed that workers used little empathy and tended to impose their own agenda with little regard or sensitivity to issues which had been raised by the parent. The authors suggest that confrontation appeared to have been used in an attempt not to collude with service users. They concluded that this may also reflect a wider systemic problem in that workers are left with little guidance or support in terms of how they combine partnership and protection or develop the micro-skills for more effective interaction with parents in such difficult circumstances.

Reflect upon the themes and discussion points raised in this chapter so far and consider the following practice-based vignette where an over preoccupation with physical health risk factors is at the expense of exploring other aspects of Mark's situation.

CASE STUDY: MORE THAN JUST A DRUG USER

Mark was a 35-year-old man who had been referred to a specialist drugs and alcohol agency by his GP. His doctor had become concerned by the escalation of Mark's alco-hol use following the sudden death of his partner 12 months ago. Following her death Mark had become the sole carer of their three children aged 10, 7 and 5 years. Although not drinking excessively high daily amounts of alcohol, the GP was concerned that Mark's drinking would continue to increase if the underlying emotional issues were not addressed.

A relatively inexperienced worker new to this area of work undertook the initial assessment. Very quickly into the session the worker became very preoccupied with information gathering at the expense of really listening to Mark's story. The worker wanted to know the exact daily amounts Mark was drinking, when, the precise pattern of his alcohol consumption and whether Mark experienced physical withdrawals. He provided much information on safe drinking amounts. During the assessment Mark also revealed that he also smoked a small amount of cannabis during the week. The worker quickly focused on this with questions about the amounts he drank in conjunc-tion with cannabis and whether Mark understood about the effects of potentiation which he then proceeded to explain at length. ➔

➜

It was clear that Mark was concerned about his drinking and stated that he felt that having to see the worker was an admission of failure. He said that he had been very embarrassed about talking to his GP who had also been his partner's doctor up until her death. At two points during the assessment, Mark became tearful when talking about losing his partner and how much he and the children missed her. The worker did not respond or acknowledge this emotional content of Mark's story and indeed looked very uncomfortable when Mark became upset. Mark also tried to explain how he had provided for his children to the best of his ability, that he had always managed to get the children to school on time and was learning how to cook decent meals for them. Again, none of this was acknowledged by the worker who kept turning the conversation back to questions about alcohol intake and focusing on aspects of physical health.

Mark did not keep the follow-up appointment made for him and the agency closed his case. Later the GP contacted the agency to inform them Mark had made a suicide attempt.

CHALLENGE

■ What are your thoughts about how the worker dealt with Mark?

■ How could the worker have dealt with this situation differently?

■ How might the worker have addressed Mark's feelings and the emotional content of his situation?

Inadvertently this practitioner has neglected the key principle of person-centred practice which is to forge an effective working alliance where the service user feels able to explore the many complex and often interrelated aspects of his situation. This can easily happen with the over-zealous or novice practitioner. It is common for workers to want to focus on the service user's substance use and related difficulties, while the service user's priority may be to discuss a wider range of concerns. This has been termed the 'premature-focus trap' (Miller and Rollnick, 1991: 69).

The message is to start with the service user's concerns and agenda rather than those of the practitioner. In the above situation, in Mark's mind, the substance use may be a relatively small part of the picture and it will be important to acknowledge this within the practitioner-service user relationship. In a similar vein, it is also important for practitioners to acknowledge and be sensitive to conflicting and fluctuating degrees of motivation on the service user's part as well as recognise that ambivalence is often central to any process of changing behaviour. It is this area which will now be discussed.

Service users' motivation and readiness to engage in change

It is important for practitioners to have a clear understanding of motivation as a psychological process and framework to assess readiness to make any changes in their use of substances. Motivational enhancement therapy has been discussed by Gardner (2004) and seeks to mobilise the individual's own resources to bring about change. The practitioner's role is to create a supportive, collaborative environment where problems can be explored and motivation grows. Central to this approach is a model of change (Prochaska and DiClemente 1982) which seeks to explain why and how people make changes either on their own or with the practitioner's help. They describe a series of changes that a person goes through in the process of changing a problem:

■ *Precontemplation*: Where the user does not even contemplate having a prob-lem or needing to make a change. Such individuals may be identified during a routine medical examination for example. Frequently people in this stage do not engage with services or only attend because they are under some pres-sure to do so.

■ *Contemplation*: once there is an awareness of the problem, the individual may enter a period characterised by ambivalence. The contemplator may simultaneously want and not want to make changes.

■ *Determination*: the individual is making up their mind to do something about the problem. In this stage, a typical statement may be 'I've got to do something about my drinking'. It has been described as a 'window of opportunity' where the person enters in to action or reverts back to contemplation.

■ *Action*: Where the substance user engages in particular actions intended to bring about change and acts on their plans.

■ *Maintenance*: The task is to sustain the change achieved by previous action and prevent relapse.

■ *Relapse*: Where the task is to start around the cycle without becoming stuck in the relapse stage (a lapse may not be a full relapse).

Table 6.1 builds on Miller and Rollnick's (1991: 18) work and provides exam-ples using alcohol and drug misuse to help the practitioner match their inter-vention to the substance user's position on the cycle of change.

The same authors also have developed Motivational Interviewing as a set of techniques to assist the process of change. A non-directive reflective style on the practitioner's part is advocated with its defining features including the following:

■ cognitive discrepancy – to augment the discrepancy between the client's current and desired behaviours

Table 6.1 Working with change: service user readiness and worker task

Stage on the model of change	Worker task	An example for practice
Pre-contemplation:	Raise doubt – increase the user's perception of risks and problems associated with current behaviour.	'Let us talk a little more about some of the implications for your general health and well-being which may follow from your current level of drinking.'
Contemplation:	Tip the balance – evokes reasons to change, risks of not changing.	'You say that your partner is the most important person to you but that she will leave you unless you stop taking amphetamines. I'm wondering then where that leaves you now in relation to your drug use …'
Determination:	Help user determine the best course of action to take in seeking change	'It sounds as though you've made up your mind to reduce the amount of alcohol you're drinking? Perhaps it would be useful to look in more detail at some of the options you've talked about.'
Action:	Help the user to take steps towards change	'Ok you said that you'd like to come to one of the support groups. Let's list some of the things that need to be sorted including child care and who's available to help you with the children to make that possible.'
Maintenance:	Help the user identify and use strategies to prevent relapse	'It seems that you've been doing a lot of things to help yourself stay off cannabis. It might now be useful to write down and firm up on the strategies you've been using to help you keep on track …'
Relapse:	Help user review stages of contemplation, determination and action without becoming stuck or demoralised because of relapse.	'OK so you had a drink over the weekend and feel bad. Let's look at that and then go back over some of the reasons why you said it was important for you to stop drinking …'

- a non confrontational style
- recognizing that ambivalence is a natural part of any process of change
- rolls with resistance
- instillation of hope
- self esteem and self efficacy are central to making positive changes. (Miller and Rollnick 1991: 32–4)

Towards a more holistic assessment: a complex practice context, risk and the responsible practitioner

'When people take any substance a complex relationship comes into play' (Allan 2010: 144). As has been shown, understanding an individual's substance use involves a careful consideration and exploration of four cornerstones – the substance user as an individual, the substance itself, the environment and, finally, the individual practitioner's degree of knowledge, experience and attitudes towards substance use and those who misuse substances.

The models outlined above are particularly helpful as they walk alongside the person misusing substances rather than trying to impose a solution upon them. Effectively the individual who misuses substances carries out a daily cost/benefit analysis (or risk assessment) of their situation, balancing the benefits (the feeling they get from taking the substance or the negation of painful withdrawal symptoms) against the costs or risks (to the person's health, relationships, finances, employment etc.). In order to work effectively with someone misusing substances, the practitioner has to recognise the motivational ambivalence that informs giving up a substance that has become a physical or psychological necessity, and the fact that this may take several attempts, and may indeed never be achieved.

It is important for practitioners to be able to conduct a competent and effective assessment of substance use and related problems. Some of the reasons why practitioners should develop their assessment skills include:

- enhancing the quality of information gathering

- making assessment an empowering process

- understanding the determination of eligibility

- providing access to solutions and the most suitable services offering sensitivity and support at a time that is often stressful. (Whittington 2007: 17)

Given the complexity and multifaceted nature of substance misuse, it is important that practitioners understand that assessment can serve several purposes and functions. The extent to which practitioners adopt a particular assessor role(s) will be dependent on their particular practice context and setting, as discussed by Whittington (2007):

Five purposes of assessment – the interest or goal for which assessor is agent

1. Individual and public protection: for the risk assessor the purpose is the protection of individual service users and carers, other members of the public and staff.
2. Service user and carer needs: 'Traditional professional' – purpose is in line with a person-centred approach focusing on needs, expectations, problems and solutions, weaknesses and strengths mediated by the practitioner's professional judgment.
3. Service user and carer representation: Advocate practitioners need to assess the role they are required to play and judge whether they should act as an advocate.
4. Agency function, policy and priorities: Agency representative-role is characterised by the task of implementing agency policy and priorities or 'agency function' determined by boundaries such as eligibility criteria.
5. Other professions or agencies: Proxy when the practitioner is engaged in assessment to provide information to facilitate others' decision making such as courts of law. (Adapted from Whittington 2007: 25)

As we have seen the tension between autonomy and protection is a key feature of the helping professions and is not easily reconciled. Some of these debates are indeed crystallised when working in the field of substance use (Stalker 2003). Consider the aspect of coercion within the criminal justice system. Coerced treatment for substance misuse in the form of Drug Treatment and Testing orders was introduced with the 1998 Crime and Disorder Act for those offenders with a propensity to misuse drugs to receive treatment supported by specialist drug agencies (Goodman 2009: 41). This is further explored by Pycroft (2010) who highlights how a criminal justice system approach appears to be completely at odds with the nature of addiction:

> although drug use may involve choice, when that use becomes 'addictive behaviour' we are faced with a system of impaired control and relapse as a centrally defining feature. Within this complex biopsychosocial paradigm responsibility becomes an aspiration and not a given ... If a person has a problem such as addiction and is seeking to overcome it, then like any major change in life it is something that may take time and require encouragement rather than condemnation. (Pycroft 2010: 130)

The practice and policy landscape continues to change with accompanying changes to how services are delivered and provided.

> Balancing service user risk taking, rights, autonomy and empowerment with issues of protection in ... a context of limited resources, increasing public scrutiny and fear of professional litigation is complex. (Mitchell and Glendinning 2008: 4)

Similarly, the notions of capacity and incapacity feature prominently within debates with 'the assumption that the State does not seek to intervene unnecessarily in the life of its citizens and will therefore not interfere with the choices anyone makes provided they are lawful choices' (Hothersall *et al.* 2008: 59).The continued marketisation of care with its outcome-focused emphasis targeted on those most in need would suggest that 'risk' criteria and risk assessment will remain central to the practitioners' role (Fenge 2006).

Clearly, and as discussion throughout this chapter has shown, risk operates as a 'complex construct' (Stanford 2010: 1071). This demands that practitioners negotiate the often equally complex world of substance misuse with a critical, measured and evidence-informed approach. Recent research (Stanford 2010) indicates that the stance adopted by practitioners and how they identified themselves and recognised their service users strongly influenced how risk was operationalised within their practice. Stanford describes four positions, where the client or the practitioner may be seen to be 'at risk' or to pose 'a risk'. Some practice-grounded substance misuse examples have been added here to illustrate each definition:

- 'Client at risk' – 'She can't deal with a lot of areas in her life – the abuse she suffered as a child keeps coming back to haunt her so she deals with it by blotting it all out with drugs – she never feels in control of her life …'

- 'Client a risk' – 'He doesn't care what he does to get his drugs … he'll take on anybody, do anything …'

- 'Practitioner at risk' – 'If service users are intoxicated, it rings alarm bells for me. I start feeling really vulnerable and I'll always try to cut the visit short and usually don't ask as many probing questions as I would normally …'

- 'Practitioner a risk' – 'I just kept looking at them both and couldn't understand how they had got themselves into such a state through their drugs. I felt full of anger at what they were doing to the kids. In these situations it's all I can do not to have a real go at them – luckily I don't – imagine being hauled over the coals for professional misconduct …'

There is evidence that practitioners remain underconfident in their abilities to address drug and alcohol misuse effectively: 'child care workers lack sound knowledge of the effects of mental illness, drug or alcohol misuse. Respondents to the project considered that this lack of understanding came from colleagues being fearful of the unknown' (Kearney *et al.* 2003).

If as Stanford concludes, fear operates as 'an important constituent' (Stanford 2010: 1078) for defining the context within which conflicts and dilemmas were experienced and responded to, then there is some urgency to address this. Practice based on fear is not conducive to effective or informed direct work with those who use substances or with the families, carers and significant others within the substance user's wider networks.

Conclusion

Written with the non-specialist in mind, this chapter has shown the need for practitioners to adopt a critical, measured and evidenced-informed approach when working with those people who use and may misuse a range of substances. Such an approach may seem very difficult to adopt given the highly pressurised and risk-preoccupied reality of many practitioners' working lives. This chapter has, however, aimed to show how theoretically and research informed practitioners who are also able to exercise responsibility for scrutinising their personal and professional values are better placed to undertake effective and non-stigmatising practice.

Discussion has highlighted a number of ways in which vulnerability may feature in substance users' lives and the ways in which they may become subject to differing and competing agendas including those of the criminal justice system, health and social services. It is a complex task for practitioners to balance risks and rights whilst recognising and working within the limits of personal and professional responsibilities.

In the ideal world, as Pycroft observes, to achieve the possibility of change the full range of interventions should be available from harm reduction through to psychological interventions to build self-efficacy and self-esteem as well as tackling social context factors such as housing and employment. Given the current and rapidly changing practice context, he offers a timely incitement to see the world through the substance user's eyes: 'This is a complicated world even for the professionals engaged in it, so how much more confusing can it be for the anxious and vulnerable service users?' (Pycroft 2010: 114).

Useful further resources

www.talktofrank.com/ – providing clear and accessible information about drugs, their actions and side effects targeted at young people.

www.drugscope.org.uk/ – Drugscope is the leading independent centre of expertise on drugs and the national membership organisation for the drug field.

www.nta.nhs.uk – National Treatment Agency for Substance Misuse provides information and research briefings on treatment outcome findings.

References

Advisory Council on the Misuse of Drugs (ACMD) (2006) *Pathways to Problems; Hazardous Use of Tobacco, Alcohol and Other Drugs by Young People in the UK and Its Implications for Policy.* London: Advisory Council on the Misuse of Drugs.
Allan, G. (2010) Substance use: what are the risks? In S. Hothersall and M. Maas-Lowit (eds), *Need, Risk and Protection in Social Work Practice.* Exeter: Learning Matters, Ch. 10.

Augoustinos, M. (1998) Social representations and ideology: towards the study of ideological representations. In U. Flick (ed.), *The Psychology of the Social*. Cambridge: Cambridge University Press, 156–69.

Burr, V. (1996) *An Introduction to Social Constructionism*. London: Routledge.

Butt, T. and Parton, N. (2005) Constructive social work and personal construct theory: the case of psychological trauma. *British Journal of Social Work*, 35(6): 793–806.

Cemlyn, S. (2008) Human rights and Gypsies and Travellers: an exploration of the application of a human rights perspective to social work with a minority community in Britain. *British Journal of Social Work*, 38: 153–73.

Chein, I. (1969) Psychological functions of drug use. In H. Steinberg (ed.), *Scientific Basis of Drug Dependence*. London: Churchill Livingstone.

Crome, I. and Chambers, P., with Frisher, M., Bloor, R. and Roberts, D. (2009) *SCIE Research Briefing 30: The Relationship between Dual Diagnosis: Substance Misuse and Dealing with Mental Health Issues*. London: SCIE.

Curran, V. and Drummond, C. (2007) Psychological treatments of substance misuse and dependence. In D. Nutt, T. Robbins, G. Stimson, M. Ince and A. Jackson (eds), *Drugs and the Future: Brain Science, Addiction and Society*. London: Academic Press.

Duras, M. (1990) 'Alcohol' in *Practicalities*. London: Flamingo.

Edwards, G. (2004) *Matters of Substance: Drugs, Is Legalization the Right Answer? Or the Wrong Question?* London: Penguin Books.

Fenge, L.-A. (2006) Community care: assessing needs, risks and rights. In K. Brown (ed.), *Vulnerable Adults and Community Care*. Exeter: Learning Matters.

Fischer, J., Jenkins, N., Bloor, M., Neale, J. and Berne, L. (2007) *Drug User Involvement in Treatment Decisions*. York: Joseph Rowntree Foundation.

Forrester, D. and Harwin, J. (2006) Parental substance misuse and child care social work: findings from the first stage of a study of 100 families. *Child and Family Social Work*, 11: 325–35.

Forrester, D., McCambridge, J., Waissbein, C. and Rollnick, S. (2008) How do child and family social workers talk to parents about child welfare concerns? *Child Abuse Review*, 17: 23–35.

Gardner, S. (2004) The role of the practice counsellor in substance misuse treatments. In N. Heather and T. Stockwell (eds), *The Essential Handbook of Treatment and Prevention of Alcohol Problems*. Chichester: John Wiley and Sons, Ch. 9.

Goodman, A. (2009) *Social Work with Drug and Substance Misusers*. Exeter: Learning Matters.

Gossop, M., Marsden, J., Stewart, D. and Kidd, T. (2003) The National Treatment Outcome Research Study (NTORS): 4–5 year follow-up results. *Addiction*, 98(3), 291–303.

Griffiths, R. and Pearson, B. (1988) *Working with Drug Users*. London: Wildwood House.

Gurney, A. (2000) Risk-taking. In M. Davies (ed.), *The Blackwell Encyclopaedia of Social Work*. Oxford: Blackwell.

Hothersall, S. J., Maas-Lowit, M. and Golightly, M. (2008) *Social Work and Mental Health in Scotland*. Exeter: Learning Matters.

Ife, J. (2001) *Human Rights and Social Work: Towards Rights Based Practice*. Cambridge: Cambridge University Press.

Kearney, P., Levin, E. and Rosen, G. (2003) *Alcohol, Drug and Mental Health Problems: Working with Families*. SCIE report 2.

Kelly, G. (1955) *The Psychology of Personal Constructs*. New York: Norton & Co.

Koubel, G. and Bungay, H. (2009) *The Challenge of Person-centred Care*. London: Palgrave Macmillan.

Loughran, H., Hohman, M. and Finnegan, D. (2010) Predictors of role legitimacy and role adequacy of social workers working with substance-using clients. *British Journal of Social Work*, 40(1): 239–56.

Lupton, D. (1999) *Risk*. London: Routledge.

Macdonald, D. and Patterson, V. (1991) *A Handbook of Drug Training*. London: Routledge.

McKellar, S. and Coggans, N. (1997) Responding to family problems, alcohol and substance misuse. *Children and Society*, 11: 53–9.

Miller, W. and Rollnick, S. (1991) *Motivational Interviewing: Preparing People for Change*. New York: Guilford Press.

Mitchell, W. and Glendinning, C. (2008) Risk and adult social care: identification, management and new policies. What does UK research evidence tell us? *Health, Risk and Society*, 10(3): 297–315.

Muir, M. (2010) Serious Case Review: Executive Summary Child T. Manchester Safeguarding Children Board, available at: www.nspcc.org.uk/inform/research/reading (accessed 25 July 2011).

Munro, E. (2011) *The Munro Review of Child Protection: Interim Report, The Child's Journey*. London: Department for Education.

National Treatment Agency for Substance Misuse (2006) *Models of Care for Treatment of Adult Drug Users*. London: National Treatment Agency.

O'Connor, L., Cecil, B. and Boudini, M. (2009) Preparing for practice: an evaluation of an undergraduate social work 'Preparation for Practice' module. *Social Work Education*, 28(4): 436–54.

Ofsted (2010) *Learning Lessons from Serious Case Reviews 2009–2010*. Available at: www.ofsted.gov.uk/publications/100087

Parsloe, P. (ed.) (1999) *Risk Assessment in Social Care and Social Work*. London: Jessica Kingsley.

Prochaska, J. O. and DiClemente, C. (1982) Transtheoretical therapy: toward a more integrated model of change. *Psychotherapy: Theory, Research and Practice*, 19: 276–88.

Pycroft, A. (2010) *Understanding and Working with Substance Misusers*. London: Sage.

Shaw, S., Cartwright, A., Spratley, T. and Harwin, J. (1978) *Responding to Drinking Problems*. London: Croom-Helm.

Shephard, A. (1990) *Substance Dependency: A Professional Guide*. Birmingham: Venture Press.

Smale, G., Tuson, G., Biehal, N. and Marsh, P. (1993) *Empowerment, Assessment, Care Management and the Skilled Worker*. London: HMSO.

Smale, G., Tuson, G. and Statham, D. (2000) *Social Work and Social Problems: Working towards Social Inclusion and Social Change*. Basingstoke: Palgrave.

Stalker, K. (2003) Managing risk and uncertainty in social work: a literature review. *Journal of Social Work*, 3: 211–33.

Stanford, S. (2010) 'Speaking back' to fear: responding to the moral dilemmas of risk in social work practice. *British Journal of Social Work*, 40(4): 1065–80.

Thompson, N. (2000) *Theory and Practice in Human Services*. Basingstoke: McGraw-Hill.

Tindall, B. (1997) People with learning difficulties: citizenship, personal developement and the management of risk. In H. Kemshall and J. Pritchard (eds), *Good Practice in Risk Assessment and Risk Management*, Vol. 2: *Protection, Rights and Responsibilities*. London: Jessica Kingsley.

Whittington, C. (2007) *Assessment in Social Work: A Guide for Learning and Teaching*. London: SCIE.

CHAPTER 7

Taking Relationships into Account in Mental Health Services

Janet Melville-Wiseman

Introduction

There is an imperative for professionals to understand and address issues of risk in mental health care. However, this has largely been predicated on inquiries into high profile cases where physical harm was the dominant factor (Prins 2004); policy developments in response to public concerns about the relationship between violence and mental ill health (Department of Health 1998; Mental Health Act 2007); and the continuing preoccupations in mental health services with the medical model of care and treatment (Repper and Perkins 2003). Service providers and mental health professionals are also well informed about models and methods of assessment and management of physical manifestations of risk as these consistently form part of ongoing pre- and post-registration training for such professionals (Department of Health 2008). However, additional forms of risk associated with mental health needs and key relationships are less well understood. These needs can be complex and multidimensional and so there is a similar imperative to establish a robust and holistic approach to the assessment and management of them.

This chapter offers readers an opportunity to consider different aspects of relational risk, rights and responsibility when working with people with mental health needs. It draws on the social model of mental health and also on the principles of the recovery model (Repper and Perkins 2003). It aims to draw attention to previously little explored multiple dimensions of relational risk which can be understood in terms of risk within and to important relationships including family relationships, past and present; and risks within relationships in mental health services. The chapter explores the nature and significance of sustaining relationships for people with mental health needs (Repper and Perkins 2003; Wallcraft 2005); the importance of understanding past experiences of relational violence and abuse in the lives of particularly women with mental health needs (Williams 1996; Read and Fraser 1998; Agar and Read 2002); and the experiences of relational abuse between service users and other service users and service users and professionals in the mental health system (Garrett and Davis 1994; Williams and Keating 1999; Jackson 2006; Melville-Wiseman 2008). In addition the chapter examines the need to balance issues such as the needs of children where a parent has mental health needs; the needs of people with mental health needs to be supported to maintain important relationships, including with their children, during periods of admission to hospital; and the need for practitioners to take account of the long-term impact of interpersonal violence and abuse in the lives of women with mental health needs, including the need to be able to take a sexual abuse history.

This chapter also explores the challenges for professionals when people with mental health needs are harmed when receiving mental health services. This can be harm perpetrated by other service users (Williams and Copperman 2002; MIND 2004) or by professionals providing care and treatment (Williams and Keating 1999; Melville-Wiseman 2008). In that context there is increasing evidence that mental health practitioners across all disciplines form a significant number of referrals to professional regulatory bodies in terms of inappropriate relationships or sexual boundary violations with service users (GSCC 2008; MIND 2004). This is an issue which impacts primarily on the mental health and well-being of the victim, the victim's family and other relationships, the perpetrator and their family, and other service users, colleagues and service providers where the abuse occurs.

LEARNING OUTCOMES

By the end of the chapter you should have developed your understanding of:

- The need to consider relational needs and risks

- A complex range of issues that relate to the assessment of relational needs and risks

- Barriers to considering relational needs and risks

- Tools to support the assessment of relational needs and risks

- The potential positive impact of developing holistic practice in this area.

Overview of key evidence

There has been growing evidence of the need to think about relational issues in mental health services. This evidence usually focuses on a single dimension of relational needs and risk such as the impact of past experiences of relational violence and abuse in the lives of particularly women with mental health needs (Williams 1996; Read and Fraser 1998; Agar and Read 2002); the nature and significance of sustaining relationships for people with mental health needs (Repper and Perkins 2003; Wallcraft 2005); the impact of caring on the mental health needs of women in particular and attitudes to women with mental health needs who are mothers (Onwumere *et al.* 2008); lack of progress on gender sensitive services and related to that, relational abuse between services users when using services and inappropriate relationships between vulnerable mental health service users and mental health professionals (Garrett and Davis 1994; Williams and Keating 1999; Jackson 2006; Melville-Wiseman 2008). People who use mental health services need aspects of relational needs and risks taken into account in a holistic way.

Relationships and mental health

Relationships that are positive and sustaining are protective factors for all of us in terms of our emotional and psychological well-being. This is true across the lifespan and across gender, ethnicity, sexuality and economic status. However, negative experiences in relationships past or present can be a significant causal factor in terms of either current or future mental health problems. This suggests that a key dimension of the assessment process in mental health services should include an assessment of the nature and quality, both positive and negative, of past and current relationships, the risks and needs associated with those relationships and the impact on those relationships of the current mental health issues or use of services. However, this can be problematic especially in the context of administrative divisions for the delivery of services. For example, social work is usually delivered from teams working with children, adults or people with mental health needs. Each team is focused on the needs of their individual service user group and with often competing priorities for intervention. For example, in the case of a mother with a young child, the child's needs may be paramount but does that mean that the mother struggling to cope with her child as well as her mental health needs does not have any important needs of her own including in relation to her child? In assessing the child's needs how much weight is given to helping them to understand their mother's mental health needs as opposed to protecting the child from those mental health issues? If this important work is to be carried out who should do that and how should it be coordinated? The mother's social worker, because of their specialist practice, probably has the most expertise in terms of understanding mental health needs but the child's social worker, because of their specialist practice, may have the greatest expertise in terms of communicating with a child of that age. A mental health nurse in an in-patient setting may see a child regularly during visits and so they may be the best person to get to know the child and answer their questions. However, the segregation and congregation of people into age or problem focused services with associated specialist professionals can only support a holistic approach to key relationships if professionals are committed to working together (Sheehan 2004).

The fragmentation of services into these administrative service delivery groups does not reflect the relational structure of people's lives either, which usually cross age groups and needs. It therefore has the potential to reinforce the fragmentation and disintegration of key relationships within families or social networks and thus marginalise relational needs and risks. This lack of a systemic approach can lead to potentially mental health affirming relationships being unnecessarily severed and those relationships that may pose a risk to an individual's mental health not being thoroughly assessed. Similarly when inter-familial relational risk is not assessed in its full complexity, risk from members of such families with mental health needs will not be fully assessed and managed.

When a parent has mental health needs

Parents and particularly mothers with mental health needs have often been the focus of concern in terms of the risk that they may harm or neglect their children (Humphreys and Thiara 2003). However, whilst it is true that the majority of child violence related deaths occur in the family, and it is possible that at least one parent may have mental health needs, the rates have fallen in the UK by 70 per cent (from 203 per million to 61 per million) in the last forty years (Pritchard and Sharples 2008). Understanding and accurately assessing this risk is a crucial part of the mental health and child protection interface but this should not obscure the needs of the overwhelming majority of children and parents to be supported to continue to have meaningful relationships when mental health needs are present. The accurate assessment of any risk of physical harm to children includes knowing when it is likely to be a real and imminent risk, when there is a possible risk and when there is little or acceptable risk. Very few people with mental health needs are permanently unwell and even fewer pose a permanent risk. It is therefore a key role to assess how relationships between parents and their children can be both kept safe and sustained. However, there is evidence that the existence of children in the family of a person who uses mental health services is not even routinely recorded by those services (Slack and Webber 2007). In addition Agar and Read (2002) found that when people with mental health needs reported current abuse to mental health professionals in in-patient settings that abuse was not reported to the correct authorities even if children were left at risk.

Women and caring

The caring roles that women often undertake in relation to children and others are often studied from the perspective of the burden this caring can bring and the mental health implications of taking on such roles (Department of Health 2008). However, there is also evidence that undertaking such roles can have a mental health enhancing effect. This can include giving a feeling of increased self-worth and improved relationships between the care receiver and care giver (Onwumere *et al.* 2008). However, this dimension is rarely considered in mental health assessments and particularly when the person cared for is a child.

Many women who have mental health needs are also mothers and it is crucial that mental health services understand the relational needs and risks for both the mother and her child or children (Department of Health 2003). This includes the need for a mother to be supported to care for her child during a period of mental ill health; the need for the child to be cared for or to maintain contact with their mother during a period of mental ill health of the mother; the need for the child to be supported to understand the mother's mental health needs; the need for the caring role that some children will take on to be recognised; the need for access to community support such as Sure Start to be prioritised; the need for services to work together to plan for the relational needs and risks and the need for mental health services to provide child friendly services where mothers can be supported to stay with their children whilst receiving treatment. The *Women's Mental Health Strategy Implementation Guidance* (Department of Health 2003) also drew attention to the fact that although Social Services Children and Families teams have a key child protection role in this scenario they also have a role to support the welfare of children including the maintenance of their relationships with their mothers. They also need to take account of the additional distress a mother will feel during a period of ill health if her children need to be taken into the care system. If it is necessary for a child to become 'Looked After' during a period of their mother's ill health this plan needs to include how the child will maintain contact with their mother and how they will be prepared for her return to the full-time caring role if appropriate. However, discharge planning for the mother often only considers the relational needs of both mother and child where there may be concerns of ongoing risk to the child (Sheehan 2004).

More recently services have developed whereby treatment is now delivered in the home environment where possible to prevent the need for admission to hospital. However, if this is implemented in a 'one size fits all' approach it may fail to take account of the complexity of relational needs and risks in the mother and child relationship. Khalife *et al.* (2009) found that whilst mothers seemed to respond better to being treated at home, children often preferred their mother to be treated in hospital in order to give them some respite from their caring role. However, this suggests that services should be providing better choices and more comprehensive services for both mothers and their children than simply treatment at home or treatment in hospital.

======== **CHALLENGE** ========

Draw the diagram in Figure 7.1 for yourself. Add the people (including children) with whom you have regular contact. Highlight the ones that you feel sustain your emotional or mental well-being and the ones that cause you stress or worry. Add each person under each category by name in the circles.

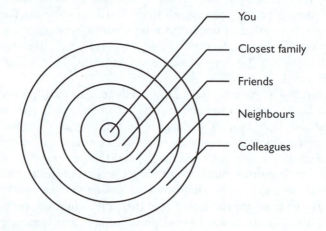

You

Closest family

Friends

Neighbours

Colleagues

Figure 7.1 Plotting key relationships

Source: Adapted from Sunderland Children's Services (2009) *Service user perspectives on the 'ethically good practitioner'.* Workshop held as part of 'Social welfare ethics: Learning professional wisdom, courage and compassion' Conference. Durham University 15th May 2009

Now imagine that you no longer have contact with each person. Cross each one out and think about what that would mean to you and what impact it would have on you and them until there is just you left.

If someone is admitted to a psychiatric ward it will mean them moving out of their home and it is likely to be some distance from their usual community. They are likely to have much less contact or no contact with all of these people. They may be rejected by some of these people who do not understand the nature of their mental ill health or who may be influenced by current stigma. If they are children they may not understand why their parent or sibling has gone away and not know how to ask questions about it.

======== **CHALLENGE** ========

■ How can practitioners help service users to maintain their important relationships?

■ What are the particular needs of children in terms of being helped to understand if a parent is admitted to hospital with mental health needs?

■ How would you explain mental illness to a child of five, a child of eight, a child of twelve, or a child of sixteen?

■ How would you challenge any stigma?

The mental health implications of experiences of violence and abuse

The medical model of mental ill health leads us to try to understand symptoms of an illness and find the best treatment to cure it or alleviate those symptoms. However, alongside that, the social model requires us to understand the range of past experiences, including relationships, and environmental factors that may have influenced either the development of mental ill health or vulnerability to mental ill health. However, this is often confused with understanding psychodynamic approaches to the quality of early attachment experiences in relationships with primary care givers. It is often under-recognised that past experiences of violence and abuse are particularly significant, with as many as 48 per cent of women who use mental health services reporting that they had suffered sexual abuse in their childhood and 48 per cent physical abuse in childhood (Agar and Read 2002). The impact of such experiences can be varied and experiences of violence in childhood are a particular causal factor of mental ill health in women especially when it has occurred in the context of familial relationships (Humphreys and Thiara 2003). However, we also know that women who have experienced violence and abuse, and who subsequently use mental health services, do not feel that the significance of these past experiences in relationships is understood by practitioners (Williams and Copperman 2002; Humphreys and Thiara 2003).

In their study, Agar and Read (2002) found that mental health professionals routinely ignore disclosures of sexual abuse even when it is a very clear case of criminal activity. The evidence they found included the fact that 46 per cent of service users in their sample of 200 community mental health team files reported that they had disclosed to their worker, sexual or physical abuse as children or adults. This was in contrast to the fact that the researchers only found evidence of such disclosure in just over a third of files and a similar number in treatment plans. It was also found that only 22 per cent received any abuse focused therapy. The study also concludes that a history of abuse is more likely to be ignored if the professional was male and a psychiatrist. However, the reluctance to ask direct questions about abuse histories cannot be justified by concerns about the potential to 'open a can of worms' when people who use services regard these experiences as key to understanding their mental health needs and therefore key to their recovery. Agar and Read (2002) also found that when service users were directly asked by the professional assessing them if they had any experiences of violence and abuse, an 82 per cent disclosure rate was achieved compared to only an 8 per cent disclosure rate when not directly asked. When service users were asked about the connection between their past experiences of abuse and their current mental health needs 69 per cent felt there was a significant connection. However, only 17 per cent thought that staff thought there was a connection (Agar and Read 2002). As stated above the study found that there were no examples of ongoing abuse being reported to the appropriate legal authorities even if it was current and posing a potential risk to the service user or others (Agar and Read 2002).

These issues have been addressed by the *Gender and Women's Mental Health Implementation Guidance, Section 8, Violence and Abuse* (Department of Health

2003), revised guidance to the Care Programme Approach (Department of Health 2008), and more recently by the National Mental Health Development Unit (2010a) review of progress to date. However, in their recent guidance on how to address issues of sexual abuse for people with mental health needs the National Mental Health Development Unit recognises that at present there is wide variation in both local implementation and professional competence (National Mental Health Development Unit 2010b).

Consider the following case study.

CASE STUDY

Josie is 22. As a 10-year-old child she was made subject to a care order as a result of persistent sexual abuse at the hands of her stepfather. Her mother was angry that Josie disclosed this and did not support her daughter. Instead she supported her husband and as a result was not permitted to have very much contact with Josie during the rest of her childhood. Once in care Josie found it difficult to settle. She had been left with low self-esteem and found it difficult to trust either men or women who cared for her. She would often have nightmares about the abuse and often ran away and missed school. She was referred to a psychologist but found the sessions too painful. She eventually left care and was referred to a housing scheme for people with mental health needs. She has a care worker, Ellie, who has worked with her for four years now and who she likes and trusts. Ellie has never discussed the abuse with Josie but has supported her with managing her money and daily living skills. She also takes Josie shopping once a week to buy food and they usually stop and have a coffee and chat. Josie also has a boyfriend who is a mental health service user with a history of self-harm relating to his own experiences of childhood abuse. In the last few years she has struggled with depression and self-harm. In recent weeks Josie's depression has become worse and she has agreed to informal admission to hospital. This is linked to the recent disclosure by her older sister that she too was sexually abused by their stepfather.

CHALLENGE

Consider the case of Josie.

- Identify the key relationships in her life. Which ones are positive and likely to support her recovery from depression? Which ones are negative or likely to exacerbate her depression? Which relationships have the potential to have either a positive or negative impact or elements of both?

- What aspect of Josie's past or present relationships might she need support with in order to recover from her current depression?

- How would you talk with her about these issues? Would you wait for her to mention the sexual abuse or would you ask her a direct question about it?

The case of Josie presents many challenges for practitioners if her relational needs and risks are going to be taken into account. For example, a common question in an assessment, particularly when someone becomes an in-patient, is 'who is your next kin?' For Josie this question is far from straightforward and has the potential to trigger many complex feelings for her. There is no legal definition of who may be next of kin and little guidance for practitioners (National Health Service 2011). However, it is usually taken to be a close blood relative or a partner. For Josie this could mean her mother, her sister or possibly her boyfriend. But how would she decide and how could a practitioner take account of her complex relational issues when asking the question? If Josie considers her mother this may evoke painful memories of betrayal, some of which may be at the root of her current depression. If she considers her sister she may not be able to bring her to mind without it triggering the recent disclosure of her sister's own experience of abuse. Josie may also feel concerned that her sister may not want any subsequent next of kin responsibilities or that she may not be able to manage them at this point in time. Taking this into account if Josie were asked 'who would you like us to contact in an emergency?' instead of 'who is your next of kin?' her choice might be her care worker Ellie or her boyfriend.

These experiences also render women vulnerable to abuse later in life including abuse when they use mental health services (Read and Fraser 1998).

Relational risks in services

The relationships between service users and professionals have been the focus of much attention in recent years in terms of how those who are the gatekeepers and providers of services should adopt a more person-centred approach towards people who receive services (May 1995; Hewison 1995; Carey 2003; Lymberry 2005). However, the imperative at the forefront of most service provider's thinking has been how this approach may make better use of finite resources to meet those needs. However, in spite of these policy developments and the implementation of the Human Rights Act 1998 there has been little examination of the potential relational challenges this can bring at the interpersonal level. Woogara (2005) and Alexander (2006) argue that the complex nature of professional relationships and the inherent power imbalances have not thus far been addressed.

However, these new arrangements for delivering care do mean that professionals have to make significant adjustments in the way that they relate to people who use services (May 1995). The theory behind these changes was that people who use services should no longer be merely passive recipients of care but instead become active participants throughout their care pathways (Department of Health 1998, 1999). These new dimensions to the care relationship present challenges, especially in contexts where that relationship forms part of the work or therapeutic task such as in mental health services. However, May (1995) also identified that particularly in nursing practice there may be resistance to these policy initiatives where traditional constructs of the relationship may be favoured on both sides.

Another challenging dimension of relationships between professionals in mental health services and people with mental health needs is the tension created by having dual responsibilities in terms of both 'caring' and 'controlling'. It would not be unusual for a mental health professional to have to negotiate the perilous waters between being supportive and therapeutic at certain times alongside perhaps depriving the same people of their liberty whilst exercising statutory functions under the Mental Health Act 1983 (Brenner 1979; Repper and Perkins 2003). Providing a choice of worker to exercise these distinct functions may not fully answer this dilemma and resources may make this an unrealistic option. These relational tensions have not been resolved by social workers (followed by nurses and occupational therapists) becoming 'care managers' and 'care coordinators' following the implementation of the NHS and Community Care Act 1990 and evidence of this continues to emerge (Postle 2002; Carey 2003).

Social inequality

Understanding the impact of social inequality in the lives of people with mental health needs has not always been given due primacy (Williams 1996; Repper and Perkins 2003) This is particularly significant when we try to understand the relational risk and needs of the mainly women who experience abuse in mental health services (Williams and Keating 1999, 2000). However, there has been much resistance to the dangers of replicating social inequalities within services and this can make it difficult to address relational abuses perpetrated by professionals (Penfold and Walker 1984; Williams 1996; Pilgrim and Rogers 1993, 2005). The dominance of the medical model (see Introduction) inevitably marginalises the need to understand the social and relational origins of mental health needs. However, services that replicate power imbalances also make it difficult to challenge abuse that is perpetrated by professionals (Williams and Keating 1999).

Relational power imbalances in mental health services

Relationships between mental health professionals and people who use services has been the focus of much research but in very specific areas such as how to make the relationship therapeutic (O'Brien 2001) or how to work in partnership (Biehal 2005). There is also extensive literature on how to ensure professionals or the wider community are not at risk of physical harm (Hewitt 2008). However, this has not been balanced by studies that examine the risk of professionals abusing vulnerable service users. Those that have been published have been driven by psychological therapy services with resultant pathologisation of victims (Melville-Wiseman 2008).

Relationships between professionals and people who use services differ from personal relationships in many ways but the nature and scope of these distinctions is often not fully recognised and does not feature in mainline pre-registration training of mental health professionals. These differences mean that the professional has more power, and therefore greater responsibility for keeping the relationship safe. However, it is clear from recent statistics that this is a significant problem and a significant amount of the work of regulatory bodies conduct teams (GSCC 2008). This approach whereby professionals are regulated against a set of criteria embedded in a professional code of practice may fail to capture the complex challenges of relational risks within contemporary practice.

Consider the following case study.

CASE STUDY

Brian is a 45-year-old social worker in a community mental health team that covers both urban and rural areas. He is divorced with two children who he only sees occasionally and the divorce has left him feeling alone, isolated and often miserable. However, he has recently arranged to meet another woman, Jill, through an internet dating service. He has planned to meet Jill in a pub in a local village. At work he has been working with a 23-year-old woman Cara, who has had depression for some time linked to earlier experiences of sexual abuse at the hands of her father. He has known her for over two years and they have established a good relationship. She has often said that if she had not had Brian as her social worker she might not have survived the last few years.

When Brian arrives in the pub he sees Cara over the other side of the bar. He is anxious as his new date is about to arrive. However, Cara sees Brian and comes over to him and asks if she can talk to him. She looks like she has been crying. Brian also sees a woman come in who looks like the description of the woman he is about to meet.

CHALLENGE

■ How can Brian keep his relationship with Cara safe?

■ What should he say to her when she comes over to him?

■ How can he take responsibility for the boundaries without offending Cara or spoiling their working relationship?

■ How would he explain if Jill asks who Cara is?

■ How would he explain to Cara if she asks what he is doing there?

■ How could he avoid breaching boundaries of confidentiality?

There are many ways in which professionals have the majority of the power in relationship with people who use services in spite of the new rhetoric of empowerment. This includes the professional being the gatekeeper of the resources that the service user needs; having had training and therefore acquired greater knowledge; having inside knowledge of how the system works; having personal information about the service user; usually mentally well; and not suffering from the stigma and discrimination associated with mental ill health (Repper and Perkins 2003). In addition, these distinctions may have their roots in traditional class distinctions when it was expected to show deference to a professional who 'knows best'.

In his study into the power dynamics between nurses and patients Hewison (1995) observed many relational problems such as nurses assuming a parent-like approach, including issuing orders to patients to do or to refrain from certain things. They would also issue verbal reprimands if the patient did something wrong or on the other hand be patronising and belittling towards their patients through the use of 'terms of endearment' (Hewison 1995). In this scenario the language used is designed to render the patient into a child-like position whilst the nurse assumes the parental and controlling role illustrated in this example from his research. A nurse is helping a patient to bathe and is observed to say:

I'll wash your back, there you are poppet. Give me your hand, pet, your other hand, sweetie. (Hewison 1995: 80)

In this example the nurse appears to be warm and friendly towards the patient and that is most likely to be the motivation. However, when examined more closely it is the nurse who is setting the agenda for the patient (in which order different parts of her will be washed) and who therefore has the control. It would be very difficult for the patient to protest or regain control especially as the nurse is using such language. Repper and Perkins (2003) comment that the need for patients with mental health needs to maintain control over even these short interactions with staff can have a profound impact on their ability to regain control over the rest of their lives. When the staff approach is less benign than the example above the repercussions can be wider and affect others in the same ward or setting who may be witnesses to inappropriate interactions. On psychiatric in-patient wards staff sometimes create a culture whereby they maintain control by using processes that are dehumanising or humiliating for patients. This can often have the opposite of the desired affect and in fact make patients more hostile or aggressive (Alexander 2006).

This 'them and us' culture can underpin stigma, discrimination and social exclusion within services (Repper and Perkins 2003) but to the detriment of both staff and patients. There has been increasing evidence that people who work in mental health services are an emerging group of people with their own mental health needs and cultures of fear and control within the workplace do not make it easy for them to seek the help and support they need either (Hawton *et al.* 2002; Stanley *et al.* 2006).

Sexual abuse of people who use mental health services

The National Patient Safety Agency is a National Health Service organisation established in 2001 to monitor and analyse adverse incidents involving patients in NHS care. Their statistics are obtained through a voluntary reporting system with NHS Trusts and at present this has rolled out to 50 of the 65 mental health trusts in England and Wales. In 2006 the National Patient Safety Agency published a worrying report on patient safety on mental health wards in the UK including the sexual abuse of patients (National Patient Safety Agency 2006). The data is gathered from ward staff and managers only and not directly from patients and so can be viewed as a conservative estimate of the true figures. Between 2003 and 2005, 122 incidents of a sexual nature had been reported including 19 incidents of alleged rape. Of these alleged rapes 11 were alleged to have been perpetrated by staff. However, whilst the agency did not gather data on whether these incidents were reported to the police or whether any were successfully prosecuted it does comment on a potential link between the patient's mental health needs and the allegations:

> The patient's underlying diagnosis may be a factor in such allegations and, from an examination of the narrative of these incidents, it appears that the contribution of the patient's underlying condition to the substance of the allegation was considered. (National Patient Safety Agency 2006: 38)

The figures reported above are similar to a survey conducted by Jackson (2006) who asked 44 NHS Mental Health Trusts to identify how many incidents of sexual assault on in-patient wards had been reported. In three years from 2003 to 2006 there were 300 incidents of which 76 (25 per cent) were allegedly perpetrated by staff (Jackson 2006). However, as above this study relied on evidence from cases that were reported to managers of the wards and so did not take account of incidents which were not reported or not recorded as reported.

Another study using figures from WITNESS paints a similar picture (WITNESS was a small UK charity set up to support victims of professional abuse in health and social care settings. It has now been closed but their work continues through the Clinic for Boundary Studies). However, these figures are gleaned from victims of professional sexual abuse seeking support from the organisation in a single year (2005) (Coe 2006). Psychotherapists formed the largest group (18) followed by mental health nurses (11); GPs and counsellors (10 each); care workers (9); social workers and hypnotherapists (5 each); psychiatrists (4) and gynaecologists (3). Others noted were a yoga teacher in a mental health setting, a dentist, a religious minister, a helpline volunteer and a housing officer. WITNESS welcomed contact from victims across the full spectrum of health and social care services but it is interesting to note that the majority of their referrals (59 per cent, $n = 61$) were linked to mental health professionals or those offering some kind of emotional or psychological aspect of a physical problem. In addition, two of the most high profile cases of professional sexual abuse that have led to public inquiries in recent years involved two psychiatrists, Dr Kerr and Dr Haslam (Pleming 2005).

> ### CASE STUDY
>
> Consider the case of a mental health social worker, Gerry, who is 45 and married to Rosemary who is a mental health nurse. They have three daughters – Daisy aged 10, Flora aged 12 and Naomi aged 16. Gerry has been working with a young woman Shelley who is 22 and who has a history of self-harming and depression. This is linked to earlier experiences of both physical and sexual abuse by her mother's boyfriend when Shelley was between 10 and 15 years old. Gerry has been seeing Shelley for over two years, usually at the day centre she attends, and feels that he has gained Shelley's trust. She has recently been admitted to hospital following an overdose and on discharge Gerry makes a follow-up visit to Shelley at her flat. Shelley is very distressed and asks Gerry for a hug which he gives her. He is then aware that he finds Shelley attractive and is enjoying the physical contact. The hug becomes sexual and Shelley does not push him away. They end up having sex. Two weeks later Gerry tells a colleague what happened. The colleague reports it to a senior manager and Gerry is suspended pending an inquiry. Gerry is also reported to the GSCC.

CHALLENGE

Consider the impact of this scenario on:

■ Shelley – how might it affect her mental health needs? How might it affect any future relationships with a partner and with mental health professionals?

■ Rosemary – how might her relationship with her husband be affected? What might her concerns be at this point? How might she feel towards Shelley or the colleague who reported her husband? How might her work as a mental health nurse be affected?

■ Naomi, Flora and Daisy – how might they feel and what might help them to come to terms with what has happened?

■ Gerry's colleagues – how might they respond to him being suspended and the reasons? What might their concerns be? How might the colleague who 'blew the whistle' feel right now? What did they feel before they reported Gerry?

■ Gerry – what are the implications for him and his relationships with his wife, his children, his colleagues?

■ How could this have been prevented?

Keeping relationships safe in mental health services

It is clear that there are a complex set of factors that impact on the relationships between professionals and the people they work with in mental health services. There are considerable risks given that people who have experienced relational abuses in the past will form a significant number of people who have mental health needs in later life. It is crucial that the relationships are safe as well as therapeutic. Responsibility for keeping them safe lies with the professional but is underpinned by their training, their support to carry out what is demanding work and their access to supervision that provides a safe place to look at potential problems before they become harmful. However, relational risks do not always feature as a key part of pre-registration or pre-qualifying training.

There have been different proposals for pre-qualifying registration training in relationship or boundary issues such as for social workers (Davidson 2005), medical students (White 2004), nurses (Peternelj-Taylor and Yonge 2003) and psychiatric registrars (Vamos 2001). In addition the Clear Boundaries Project (Council for Healthcare Regulatory Excellence 2008) included an education stream in its review of sexual boundary issues in health and social care. The consensus, therefore, is that specific training on relational boundary issues should be an integral part of teaching professionals how to both manage their own boundaries but also challenge poor boundary holding in colleagues.

Within the context of understanding professional relationships and boundary holding it is important to draw a distinction between what might lead to an appropriate relationship and what might constitute a good, helpful or therapeutic relationship for people with mental health needs. Where proper boundaries are not maintained vulnerable people will be harmed. However, either way their relationships will still be characterised by imbalances of power and so the challenge for the professional to form an appropriate and helpful relationship is immense.

It is also the case as we have seen above that many people with mental health needs have experienced many forms of boundary violations before they come into contact with a professional. It is therefore likely that those people will not find it easy to trust even the most boundaried professional and are likely to need to test both where the boundaries in the relationship are, whether the professional is trustworthy and whether they know how to neither over- or under-react to boundary challenges. It is often the case that people with mental health needs who need to test the boundary holding ability of a professional are often criticised for having that need. But where else should they take the aftermath of those experiences other than to the professional who is paid to help them with their problems?

Professional codes of practice may not be sufficient to help professionals work out how to apply these principles in practice. They often include principles and proscriptions against certain activity within professional relationships but they do not show registrants how to develop individual skills in this regard. They also do not give many clues about the characteristics of good professional relationships. However, in a critical analysis of professional boundaries Davidson (2005) provides an alternative framework. Instead of conceptualising professional boundaries as a straight line between appropriate behaviour and inappropriate behaviour Davidson (2005) argues that relationships should be viewed as being on a continuum from entangled on the one hand to rigid on the other and that both extremes are potentially harmful. However, in the middle is an area where there is some flexibility as opposed to a single line or crossing point between appropriate and inappropriate boundaries. Furthermore, Davidson (2005) argues that there are degrees of stepping outside of this safe balanced zone of flexibility between breaches and violations. Stepping outside of that balanced position can then lead, in the first instance, to a breach of professionals boundaries and, if taken further, to a violation of those boundaries. Professionals with 'rigid' relationships with their clients are described as ones who:

> barrel ahead with their own agenda inflexibly, condescendingly, and without attending to the unique and multifaceted needs of the client. Their lack of authenticity and sensitivity while attending to the client's needs contravenes their ethical responsibility to honour the dignity and worth of the individual. Responding rigidly exploits the client's vulnerabilities and is an abuse of the professional's position of power as it accentuates, and even exaggerates, the power differential between them. (Davidson 2005: 519)

In contrast those in 'entangled' relationships are characterised as primarily meeting their own needs in the relationship to the detriment of their client's. This can include meeting 'their own emotional, social, or physical needs through the relationship with their client, at the expense of the client' (Davidson 2005: 518).

It is this entangled position that can also lead to abusive sexual relationships between professionals and people who are vulnerable with mental health needs.

CASE STUDY

You are meeting a woman service user on your own in an interview room at work. She is telling you about a very distressing experience and is tearful. She leans forward and takes your hand. You do not feel comfortable with reciprocating or accepting this physical contact. However, you are also aware that this woman has just begun to open up to you about her distressing feelings and you wish to show empathy.

- What do you do?
- What do you say?
- Would you respond differently if the service user was not upset?

CHALLENGE

Using Davidson's model of balanced relationships (being neither rigid nor entangled but with some limited scope for flexibility) consider your answers to the above questions.

- Are they towards the rigid side or entangled side of the spectrum?
- How are these professional relationships different to personal relationships?
- What are the implications of this for people who you work with?

Conclusions

This chapter has drawn attention to some of the challenges of responding to relational risks in mental health services. These risks are not always well understood or articulated but if ignored have the potential to exacerbate the very problems that people need services to help with. Addressing these risks includes understanding the mental health implications of earlier experiences of violence and abuse; recognising that professionals have their own mental health needs which may mirror those of the people they work with; the need to understand how those experiences may impact on professional relationships from both perspectives; understanding the need to take a non-judgemental approach to the inevitable boundary testing of people who have boundaries violated in the past and understanding the need to remain balanced in responses to the relational vulnerability of people with mental health needs.

References

Agar, K. and Read, J. (2002) What happens when people disclose sexual or physical abuse to staff at a community mental health centre? *International Journal of Mental Health Nursing*, 11(2): 70–9.

Alexander, J. (2006) Patients' feelings about ward nursing regimes and involvement in rule construction. *Journal of Psychiatric and Mental Health Nursing*, 13: 543–53.

Biehal, N. (2005) Changing practice: participation, rights and community care. *British Journal of Social Work*, 23: 443–58.

Brenner, C. (1979) Working alliance, therapeutic alliance, and transference. *Journal of the American Psychoanalytic Association*, 27(S): 137–57.

Carey, M. (2003) Anatomy of a care manager. *Work, Employment and Society*, 17(1): 121–35.

Coe, J. (2006) Evidence and impact of abuse. In Council for Healthcare Regulatory Excellence, *Clear Boundaries Project: Launch of a National Network – Conference Report*. Available at: http://www.clearboundaries.co.uk/page11.htm. London: Clear Boundaries Project web (accessed 26 August 2006).

Council for Healthcare Regulatory Excellence (2008) *Learning about Sexual Boundaries between Healthcare Professionals and patients: A Report on Education and Training*. London: Council for Healthcare Regulatory Excellence.

Davidson, J. C. (2005) Professional relationship boundaries: a social work teaching module. *Social Work Education*, 24(5): 511–33.

Department of Health (1998) *Modernising Mental Health Services, Safe, Sound and Supportive*. London: Department of Health.

Department of Health (1999) *National Service Framework for Mental Health: Modern Standards and Service Models*. London: Department of Health.

Department of Health (2003) *Gender and Women's Mental Health Implementation Guidance, Section 8, Violence and Abuse*. London: Department of Health.

Department of Health (2008) *Refocusing the Care Programme Approach Policy and Positive Practice Guidance*. London: Department of Health.

Garrett, T. and Davis, J. (1994). Epidemiology in the UK. In D. Jehu (ed.), *Patients as Victims*. Chichester: Wiley.

GSCC (General Social Care Council) (2008) *Raising Standards: Social Work Conduct in England*. Available at: http://www.gscc.org.uk (accessed 10 February 2010).

Hawton, K., Simkin, S., Rue, J., Haw, C., Barbour, F., Clements, A., Sakarovitch, C. and Deeks, J. (2002) Suicide in female nurses in England and Wales. *Psychological Medicine*, 32: 239–50.

Hewison, A. (1995) Nurses' power in interactions with patients. *Journal of Advanced Nursing*, 21: 75–82.

Hewitt, J. L. (2008) Dangerousness and mental health policy. *Journal of Psychiatric and Mental Health Nursing*, 15: 186–94.

Humphreys, C. and Thiara, R. (2003) Mental health and domestic violence – 'I call it symptoms of abuse'. *British Journal of Social Work*, 33: 209–26.

Jackson, C. (2006). Out of sight. Are trusts doing enough to prevent rape and sexual assault on psychiatric wards? *Mental Health Today*, 6(7): 8–9.

Khalife, H., Murgatroyd, C., Freeman, M., Johnson, S. and Killaspy, H. (2009) Home treatment as an alternative to hospital admission for mothers in a mental health crisis: a qualitative study. *Psychiatric Services*, 60(5): 634–9.

Lymberry, M. (2005) United we stand? Partnership working in health and social care and the role of social work in services for older people. *British Journal of Social Work*, 36(7): 1119–34.

May, C. (1995) Patient autonomy and the politics of professional relationships. *Journal of Advanced Nursing*, 21: 83–7.

Melville-Wiseman, J. (2008) Pathologies or apologies? A case study of an incident of professional sexual abuse in the mental health system. Unpublished PhD thesis, University of Kent.

MIND (2004) *Ward Watch*. Available at: http://www.mind.org.uk/assets/0000/0353/ward_watch_report.pdf (accessed 10 February 2010).

National Health Service (2011) *NHS Data Model and Dictionary Version 3.* Available at: http://www.datadictionary.nhs.uk (accessed 4 February 2011).

National Mental Health Development Unit (2010a) *Working towards Women's Well-being – Unfinished Business*. Available at: http://www.nmhdu.org.uk/silo/files/working-towards-womens-wellbeing-unfinished-business.pdf (accessed 4 February 2011).

National Mental Health Development Unit (2010b) *Sexual Abuse*. Available at: http://www.nmhdu.org.uk/our-work/mhep/gender/sexual-abuse/ (accessed 4 February 2011).

National Patient Safety Agency (2006). *With Safety in Mind: Mental Health Services and Patient Safety*. Patient Safety Observatory Report 2. London: National Patient Safety Agency.

O'Brien, A. J. (2001) The therapeutic relationship: historical development and contemporary significance. *Journal of Psychiatric and Mental Health Nursing*, 8: 129–37.

Onwumere, J., Kuipers, E., Bebbington, P., Dunn, G., Fowler, D., Freeman, D., Watson, P. and Garrety, P. (2008) Caregiving and illness beliefs in the course of psychotic illness. *The Canadian Journal of Psychiatry*, 53(7): 460–8.

Penfold, P. S. and Walker, G. A. (1984) *Women and the Psychiatric Paradox*. Buckingham: Open University Press.

Peternelj-Taylor, C. A. and Yonge, O. (2003) Exploring the boundaries in the nurse–client relationship: professional roles and responsibilities. *Perspectives in Psychiatric Care*, 39(2): 55–66.

Pilgrim, D. and Rogers, A. (1993). *A Sociology of Mental Health and Illness*. Buckingham: Open University Press.

Pilgrim, D. and Rogers, A. (2005) Psychiatrists as social engineers: a study of an anti-stigma campaign. *Social Science and Medicine*, 61(12): 2546–56.

Pleming, N. (2005) *The Kerr/Haslam Inquiry*. London: The Stationery Office.

Postle, K. (2002) Working 'between the idea and the reality': ambiguities and tensions in care managers' work. *British Journal of Social Work*, 32: 335–51.

Prins, H. (2004) Mental health inquiries – 'cui bono'? In N. Stanley and J. Manthorpe (eds), *The Age of the Inquiry: Learning and Blaming in Health and Social Care*. London: Routledge.

Pritchard, C. and Sharples, A. (2008) 'Violent' deaths of children in England and Wales and the major developed countries 1974–2002: possible evidence of improving child protection? *Child Abuse Review*, 17(5): 297–312.

Read, J. and Fraser, A. (1998) Abuse histories of psychiatric in-patients: To ask or not to ask? *Psychiatric Services*, 49: 355–9.

Repper, J. and Perkins, R. (2003) *Social Inclusion and Recovery: A Model for Mental Health Practice*. London: Balliere Tindall.

Sheehan, R. (2004) Partnership in mental health and child welfare: Social work responses to children living with parental mental illness. *Social Work in Health Care*, 39(3–4): 309–24.

Slack, K. and Webber, M. (2007) Do we care? Adult mental health professionals' attitudes towards supporting service user's children. *Child and Family Social Work*, 13: 72–9.

Stanley, N., Manthorpe, J. and White, M. (2006) Depression in the profession: worker's experiences and perceptions. *British Journal of Social Work*, Advance Access published online 13 July 2006, http://bjsw.oxfordjournals.org (accessed 30 August 2006).

Vamos, M. (2001) The concept of appropriate professional boundaries in psychiatric practice: a pilot training course. *Australian and New Zealand Journal of Psychiatry*, 35: 613–18.

Wallcraft, J. (2005) Recovery from mental breakdown. In J. Tew (ed.), *Social Perspectives in Mental Health*. London: Jessica Kingsley.

White, G. E. (2004) Setting and maintaining professional role boundaries: an educational strategy. *Medical Education*, 38: 903–10.

Williams, J. (1996) Social inequalities and mental health: developing services and developing knowledge. *Journal of Community and Applied Psychology*, 6: 311–16.

Williams, J. and Copperman, J. (2002) *Mental Health Services that Work for Women: Summary Findings of a UK Survey*. Canterbury: The Tizard Centre, University of Kent.

Williams, J. and Keating, F. (1999) Abuse of adults in mental health settings. In N. Stanley, J. Manthorpe and B. Penhale (eds), *Institutional Abuse: Perspectives across the Life Course*. London: Routledge.

Williams, J. and Keating, F. (2000). Abuse in mental health services: some theoretical considerations. *Journal of Adult Protection*, 2(3): 32–9.

Woogara, J. (2005) Patients' privacy of the person and human rights. *Nursing Ethics*, 12(3): 273–87.

Interprofessional Working to Safeguard and Protect Children

Jane Greaves and Cheryl Yardley

Introduction

The issue of responsibility for safeguarding children arouses strong opinions; statutory agencies are criticised for intervening in family life, while when a child is harmed there is significant media focus on the professionals who should have 'done something' to prevent harm from occurring. Repeated inquiries into child deaths have focused attention on the need for professionals from different agencies to work together, but as we will explore in this chapter this can be a complex area; while discourses around risk are a key issue in safeguarding children (Munro 2008; Holland 2011) there are often competing professional understandings of risks and responsibilities and risk may be framed to justify a particular intervention or to contain anxiety. This chapter considers the nature of interprofessional working in safeguarding children and young people from both health and social care perspectives. There is a focus on the different professional perspectives and how these can impact on roles and responsibilities in assessing and managing risk. The current context of practice with children, young people and their families highlights the importance of multidisciplinary collaboration to safeguard and protect children (Barker 2009).

The chapter is written by authors from two different professions: one is from a background of social work with children and families, while the other has worked in public health nursing. Over the last three years we have worked together to deliver shared modules for social workers who are undertaking post-qualifying study under the General Social Care Council Post Qualifying Framework for Social Work and nurses undertaking Specialist Community Public Health Nursing training to become health visitors and school nurses registered with the Nursing and Midwifery Council. This chapter draws on our experiences of interprofessional working and learning together, both in practice and from the shared teaching.

LEARNING OUTCOMES

By the end of the chapter you should have developed your understanding of:

- The context of managing risk in safeguarding children
- Professional roles and responsibilities in managing risk
- How risk is framed to inform decision making in safeguarding
- The importance of supervision and support for those involved in safeguarding.

The context of managing risk in safeguarding children

The roles and responsibilities of different professionals in safeguarding children have changed substantially in recent years and will continue to adapt to shifting political, economic and social drivers. The term 'safeguarding' is itself contentious, linked most particularly to the substantial number of policy initiatives under the New Labour government of 1997–2010 and the ambitious aim to refocus services away from reactive child protection procedures to preventative and supportive services for families. The socio-medical model of child protection had been heavily criticised for leading to both over- and under-intervention: 'social workers were excoriated both for acting and for failing to act to protect children' (Taylor 2009: 25).

Traditionally, the medical profession has had a clear role in diagnosing abuse with the focus on 'incidents' (Corby 2005) – the collection of tangible evidence and removal of the child to safety where necessary. The document *Working Together under the Children Act 1989* (Department of Health 1991), focused on the protection of children at risk of significant harm. While the Children Act 1989 placed a statutory duty on local authorities to provide services to children deemed 'in need' under section 17 (children requiring services to enable them to maintain a 'reasonable' standard of health or development, and children with a disability), resources were concentrated on the duty to investigate concerns under section 47 and cases were 'labelled' at the point of referral leading to a significant polarisation of child protection and family support services (Parton 2006).

Two key reports (the Audit Commission 1994 and the Department of Health 1995) and media attention on the deaths of children known to agencies raised concerns about the targeting of resources. While extensive research into

child development and the impact of abuse and neglect highlighted the consequences of long-term neglect, such children were more likely to be designated
as a child 'in need' rather than 'at risk' and therefore not reach the threshold
for support. At a time of increasing unemployment and increasing numbers of
children living in poverty, in many families the lack of early support meant that
issues such as poor housing and domestic violence had a significant impact on
the health and development of the children and problems became more acute
(Kirton 2009).

The election of the Labour government in 1997 led to a change in attitudes
to state intervention and a shift from the narrow focus on 'protection' and risk
of significant harm to the broader concept of 'safeguarding' and prevention
from harm as a responsibility shared between all agencies who work with children and their families. The extensive series of policies and measures expanded
the role of the state in family life, broadened the responsibilities of all agencies
and attempted to respond to the wider range of issues which impacted on
outcomes for all children, such as unemployment and poverty, substance
misuse, antisocial behaviour and poor housing. The term safeguarding was
defined in 2002 as

> a concept that has evolved from the initial concern about children and young
> people in public care to include the protection from harm of all children and
> young people and to cover all agencies working with children their families.
> (Department of Health 2002, s1.5).

While 'risk' was still a key concept, it was not just risk of harm from abuse but
a recognition of the risks to children's future well-being owing to deprivation
and social exclusion in their early years. A few months after the inquiry into the
death of Victoria Climbié the Laming Report was published (Laming 2003),
focusing particular criticism on the organisation of child protection services and
the failure of interprofessional working to identify and respond to concerns.
The *Every Child Matters* (Department for Education and Skills 2003) initiative
followed; Laming's report (2003) was used by the government as the impetus
for a series of changes that extended the role of the state beyond investigating
and intervening where there had been abuse (Parton 2009). The focus was on
improving outcomes for all children by providing preventative services and early
intervention. These outcomes would be shared across government departments
and *Every Child Matters* and the subsequent Children Act 2004 highlighted the
importance of interprofessional working. Tools such as the Common
Assessment Framework and the Integrated Children's system were intended to
address previous concerns about poor interprofessional communication and
collaboration and to 'improve integrated working by facilitating shared understandings between practitioners ... and promoting integrated frontline services'
(Barker 2009: 30).

These initiatives have brought a number of challenges for those working with
children and families; while responsibility for safeguarding and promoting the
welfare of children is now shared among agencies and there is a wider range of

services, expectations are greater and the role of professionals has changed. The national and international preventative health care strategy for children is referred to as universal, which means providing access to services for all families with children for advice and support (Department of Health 2010; World Health Organisation (WHO) 2006). Increasingly there has been a suggestion that the expansion of universal early intervention services, such as extended school provision and Children's Centres, and the move towards integrated working, means that children who are at risk of abuse or neglect should be identified at a much earlier stage. By making family support services accessible to all and reducing the stigma of seeking support (Kirton 2009) it was hoped that more families would access early support. This applies the principle known as progressive or proportionate universalism (Marmot 2010). The focus of many early intervention and support services, however, is on early years and educational provision. While many early Sure Start local programmes initially employed qualified social workers and health professionals, budgetary constraints and staffing shortages in statutory roles impacted on the staff mix in many Children's Centres. The Children's Plan (Department for Children, Schools and Families 2007) set out the aim to engage vulnerable families through outreach work and piloting a key worker approach, but did not mention how professionals such as social workers or health visitors could be part of this initiative (Parton 2009).

At the same time measures have been introduced which have reduced professional autonomy and increased scrutiny of professionals and their decisions, through increased bureaucratic procedures and paperwork, inspection and auditing of services and performance targets (Munro 2008; Parton 2009). In response, services are using more structured assessment tools in a drive to meet the needs for certainty and record outcomes which are measurable. Both the Laming report (2003) and NHS governance structures have focused on the need for accountability and contributed to more procedural responses to risk: professional roles have changed with a move towards 'more formalized procedures of assessment and resource management' (Smith 2008: 88).

Risk assessment

Formalised models of risk assessment and safeguarding procedures may be seen as important measures both to reassure the public and to enhance the confidence of the practitioners in health and social care. Downes suggests that they can provide an 'enabling framework' but acknowledges that they may also be used as a defensive tool (1988, cited by Taylor *et al.* 2008). Within public health, Dalziel (2008) argues that the application of epidemiological principles (which sees child maltreatment within a disease model) can promote a hierarchy-driven, 'checklist' approach to child abuse, and recommends a move away from such medicalised models. However, this requires public health nurses to have confidence in their own judgement and in their understanding of the original principles of empowerment so that an open and honest approach can be re-established in working with families.

The role of the public health nurse includes offering support to all families with children as part of a universal provision of services by home visiting or in settings such as schools and children's centres. The health visitor visits new mothers and their babies and is focused on assessing the needs of the family and identifying how early intervention and prevention strategies can be utilised to minimalise risk factors that can cause significant harm to children and young people.

It has been highlighted that reactive responses to child maltreatment are inadequate and costly in human and fiscal terms (Gilbert *et al.* 2009) which explains why child maltreatment is a public health concern (WHO 2006). However, the complexity involved defies a simplistic explanation of why any attributing risk factor leads a human being to inflict harm or injury on a child. Community health services undertake needs assessment of families with children, which has been strengthened by this agreed universal approach to service delivery (Department of Health 2009). The professional role of the public health nurse in supporting family health and well-being is defined by the prevention of ill health, promotion of good health and in the protection of health, all of which require an assessment of need and complex analysis of multiple factors of vulnerability and risk. Using an ecological model approach, the WHO demonstrates the multiple factors that need to be taken into account in considering the risk of maltreatment:

■ Individual factors (of the child and or of significant others involved) e.g. sex, gender, temperament, personal history and experience of conception, birth, illness/ill health, development, disability.

■ The relationship between individuals: close relationships with family and friends that expose the individual to the possibility of perpetrating or becoming a victim of child maltreatment.

■ The community where social relationships take place: neighbourhoods, workplaces and schools but also the particular characteristics of these which may contribute to child maltreatment.

■ Societal factors involve the underlying conditions of society that influence maltreatment – such as social norms that encourage the harsh physical punishment of children, economic inequalities and the absence of social welfare safety nets. (Adapted from WHO 2006: 13)

The universal service provision by public health nurses (health visitors and school nurses) means they will often be in contact with a range of families from those who need minimal support to adapt to changes in their lives to others who do not access other health care services despite having significant family health needs. Current Coalition government policy based on 'proportional universalism' (Marmot 2010) is explained as a way of ensuring those in greater need should be offered more support.

The use of assessment of need 'tools' in the delivery of universal services have been criticised as being 'checklists' although often based on a range of indices linked to the WHO model (above). The assessment may indicate a level of risk, under the heading of vulnerability (Appleton and Cowley 2004); for example; the age of the parents, the level of family support and their own childhood experiences, the temperament of the baby and the ability of the parents to 'read' the baby's cues for attention, their use of drugs, alcohol and cigarettes, any of which may impact on the health and well-being of the child. Further assessment should consider the community in which the family live and where supportive relationships are made in addition to the prevailing societal attitudes to the care of children (see Koubel and Yardley, Chapter 4 for other models of risk assessment).

The challenge for public health nurses is to make links from the family story which is often based on stressful events. These may relate to the individual circumstances of the parent or the child, stresses which arise from the challenges of interpersonal relationships with friends and family; the environment, if housing is crowded or inadequate, may cause further stress, and pressures may also be caused by the expectations and limitations placed by society on children and parents.

Vulnerability is a core theme in the nurse's assessment of risk and has several interpretations. It could be said that all humans can be vulnerable at times of stress and change. However, all children can be considered as vulnerable because of their dependency, physical immaturity and size (individual factors) as well as the lifestyle choices made by parents and which may impact on the well-being of the child. Vulnerability may be seen therefore as a concept that relates to human defencelessness and weakness (Rose and Killien 1983).

For public health nurses their role in identifying health needs and vulnerability in families requires early intervention to prevent ill health and promote health and well-being. The expert health visitor may balance knowledge and experience of the assessment tool with an ability to collect information from the family in conversation to identify perceived risk. In comparison, the novice or support worker may resort to interrogation to ensure the task of completing the form is accomplished (see Cecil, Chapter 6 for an example of how this works).

This poses considerable challenges for the less experienced practitioner. Lack of confidence may reduce the depth of exploration that the practitioner is willing to undertake, leading to a more superficial completion of the assessment tool in question. The risk factor in this instance is contained within the lack of knowledge and training of the inexperienced practitioner to make connections between significant factors and use sophisticated communication skills to understand and clarify the family responses. In this situation the locus of the risk is located within organisational structures that allow professional activities and intervention to be reduced to a mere set of tasks that can be measured in a linear fashion. Moreover, the assessment may be seen as a 'snapshot' rather than understood as a dynamic process in which various elements shift and change over time (Taylor and Daniel 2005).

CASE STUDY

Julie and Stephen both aged 20 live in a one-bedroom rented flat on an isolated housing estate in a seaside town with their three-month-old baby, Abby. Stephen works hard as a plasterer during the week while Jane looks after Abby. Julie and Stephen enjoy the company of their friends at weekends either 'clubbing' or entertaining in the flat. Their social activities include alcohol and the recreational use of drugs. Julie's mother lives close by and they have an arrangement for Abby to stay over every weekend so the couple are able to relax and enjoy their socialising knowing Abby is cared for safely. Julie and Stephen can recover from their 'night out' and collect Abby on Sunday lunch time when they are expected for a family lunch. Abby is considered vulnerable because she is a small and dependent baby three months old.

CHALLENGE

What are the risks that Abby is being exposed to:

- by her parents' age?

- by her parents' ability to provide for her needs?

- by the environment?

- by family stress?

- by parental drugs and alcohol?

Can you also list factors within this scenario which can be considered protective for Abby?

It is crucial that the rights of Julie and Stephen, plus protective factors such as family support and their planning for the care of the baby when they are going out, are taken into account when measuring levels of risk.

The use of the term 'at risk' has been criticised as being used too generally (Parton 1997) especially where knowledge of interrelatedness of known factors in the family, environment or the child are not specified. Information is gathered about individuals and family groups to identify areas of potential need within the context of family structure and the environment that may lead to risks to the health and well-being of individuals within the family.

In the community setting identifying areas of vulnerability which underline the concept of risk requires planning, action and intervention to promote good health and prevent ill health. Specific skills are necessary to avoid an overly optimistic approach while at the same time promoting a partnership approach to empowering families. Appleton (1996) cites four roles health visitors play which highlight conflict and diversity within the role:

1. the identification of vulnerability;

2. as a support agent to the family;

3. as a referral agent to social services and other health professionals; *and*

4. as a reluctant monitor of the situation.

Lupton *et al.* (2001) refers to this dilemma for health visitors as being both supportive and monitoring for evidence of child maltreatment. This is a common theme when practitioners have to balance differing perspectives which influence their values. In essence there is a need to ensure flexibility with Lord Laming noting that '[it] is not possible to separate the protection of children from wider support to families' (Laming 2003: 6).

Professional roles and responsibilities in managing risk

CHALLENGE

▪ In safeguarding, which professionals and other workers could be involved with the child and/or family?

▪ What do you know about the training they have undertaken for their role?

▪ What are their main roles and responsibilities?

▪ How are they managed and supervised?

In considering these questions, you will have identified a wide range of professionals and support workers who work with children and families. The expansion of preventative and parenting support services such as Sure Start and Family Intervention Projects under the New Labour government's *Every Child Matters* initiative (2003) has led to an increase in the children's workforce, in particular those working in non-statutory roles, and co-location of multidisciplinary teams. As a result families may have contact with a wider range of professionals and support workers.

CHALLENGE

▪ When considering safeguarding in the challenge above, how straightforward was it to understand the different roles played by a variety of workers involved with safeguarding a child? You may reflect on the fact that families themselves may be confused about the different responsibilities of those supporting them.

▪ How do you think changes in funding as a result of Coalition policies will affect services for children and families?

One concern about a rise in interprofessional working is that it can lead to a blurring of professional roles and identities; Barker (2009) comments on the lack of clarity in *Every Child Matters* (2003) about the term 'integrated working' and how practitioners could assume that this meant a move towards a generic workforce in children's services. He highlights that one of the key factors for successful integration is that 'while there is role overlap and shared working, there is also something about each professional role that is unique' (Barker 2009: 35).

You may have identified this in thinking about the different expectations and training of professionals and others working with safeguarding, in particular considering the values and professional codes of social workers, nurses, midwives, teachers and police officers. The level of integration and collaboration may depend on the impact of different organisational cultures.

From our experience students have commented on the positive value of learning together because of how much they have learnt about each other's roles and how they carry out their jobs. For example, public health nurses have commented that they did not realise the variety of social worker roles within children and family services, while social workers feel that they have gained a greater understanding of how health workers can contribute to working with families and the wealth of knowledge and skills they have in early assessment of families and identification of risk factors to prevent child maltreatment.

Carpenter and Dickinson propose that by learning together professionals' understanding of each other's roles and responsibilities can be enhanced, and 'ultimately, through working together more effectively, this will improve the quality of care and outcomes for service users' (2008: 1). However, learning does not just take place because students are in the same learning environment; while the goal is integrated learning rather than merely 'shared listening' (Ashford and Thomas 2005), interprofessional learning can experience the same challenges as any multidisciplinary working, such as language and communication barriers. It is important that those learning together explain profession-specific terminology and recognise that they may have different understandings of some issues (Barker 2009; Barber *et al.* 2009).

Carpenter and Dickinson (2008) use Allport's contact theory (1954) to consider how people learn from each other; even if contact in an interprofessional group is positive, stereotypes can still remain because individuals are not considered representative of their group. They highlight the importance of recognising the 'superiorities and inferiorities' of each group to enhance role security. A particular issue which arises in shared learning around safeguarding is that of an apparent hierarchy of professional expertise in safeguarding. There is often deference to the expertise of social workers who hold statutory responsibility for child protection and a focus on a procedural response to issues of concern. Some practitioners working at the sharp end may assume greater levels of knowledge while the knowledge or expertise of others involved is not considered to be so relevant.

In practice, this can have a significant impact on decision making and the willingness of all those involved in interprofessional working to take responsibility and acknowledge their role in safeguarding. The concept of 'groupthink' has been applied to child protection conferences and the way in which the pressure to conform leads to consensus. Munro (2008) highlights the fact that in order to avoid conflict in group situations individuals may agree with others and be reluctant to express a different view to the 'norm'. Group members may rely on the group to take shared responsibility for a decision about risk, because of the possible consequences of any decision. As a result the decision taken may be the safest option rather than the best. In a recent training exercise with qualified health visitors a number acknowledged that they have agreed with either the social worker or the police officer in a child protection conference as they see them as having greater status in that situation.

How risk is framed to inform decision making in safeguarding

In the workplace risk assessment takes place within the context of the demands of professional bodies, the employing organisation and the legal system and the individual's ability to reflect on their personal values and beliefs. With increasing experience intuition can play an important role in decision making and practice wisdom is applied. However, the ability to articulate and reflect on this and manage the situation can be hindered by the emotional impact of safeguarding effectively and the anxiety that risk can engender.

CASE STUDY

Mary, 17 years old, and her baby daughter Ebony, aged 6 months, live in a one-bedroom basement flat in a seaside town with her partner Pete, 19 years old. Mary has moderate learning difficulties and attended a school for children with challenging behaviour until the age of 15. She met Pete in a local park while truanting from school; they have been together now for nearly 18 months. Mary and Pete have minimal contact with their own families and are living on an estate with few amenities and high levels of unemployment, vandalism and drug and alcohol abuse. Pete works in a supermarket part time and Mary looks after Ebony. They prefer to 'keep to themselves' on the estate as they do not like the people who live there.

On arriving home from work one evening Pete finds Ebony unwell and coughing and calls the 'Out of Hours' medical service; Mary says she has not wanted her bottle all day. Dr Jones visits; he is concerned as the baby seems to have been unwell for some days and he feels that the flat is cold and very untidy. Mary appears quiet and does not respond to his questions about the baby's well-being. When Dr Jones asks who supports the family Pete replies that they look out for each other and do not get on with their families or neighbours.

After leaving the flat Dr Jones contacts social services because he is so worried about the ability of the parents to care for Ebony.

═══════════════════════ **CHALLENGE** ═══════════════════════

▪ What are the individual, family and community risk factors in this situation?

▪ Why is Dr Jones concerned and what is he trying to achieve by making a referral?

▪ What may be society's views of the risks to Ebony?

▪ How do you think different professionals would perceive the risks?

In thinking about this case you will have considered the range of identified risk factors which are used in the actuarial models discussed in Chapter 2. These include Ebony's age and vulnerability, the age of her parents, where she lives, their isolation from family support, and Mary's learning disability. However, different people will place a different emphasis on each of these factors depending on their professional perspective, values and experience. You may have considered that there are a number of protective factors and that Dr Jones has only been able to make a limited assessment of the situation. From his perspective, he may feel that this is not specifically within his professional remit, but his intuition and professional norms as well as personal values lead him to feel the home circumstances and the care Ebony is receiving from her parents is worrying.

From a biomedical perspective, the health professional may believe the situation necessitates referral to an 'expert' in social services, to investigate and collect information, monitor and 'do something'; in effect alleviate the fears of the referring professional. Powell refers to this 'conveying' and escalation of fears, worries and concerns as the health professionals' emotional response to a child protection case (Powell 2007).

The emotional response can interfere with a clear and logical approach to referral and moreover impact on the success of interprofessional working as personal anxiety is projected on to other workers. It can be a strong motivation to take what may be a 'safe option' to manage risk and deflect criticism, and is framed in defensive practice. While the referral may not meet the criteria for the statutory agency to take action, the level of anxiety engendered in both the referrer and the social worker can lead to a series of defence mechanisms such as splitting and projection which compromise successful interprofessional working; these are displayed in criticisms of each other for failing to take responsibility or for not acting as expected (Taylor *et al.* 2008).

We have seen examples of this in our shared Safeguarding Children module when students have to undertake an assessed group presentation in interprofessional groups. Projection can be seen in this setting as a way of dealing with the anxiety of the exercise: if problems arise in the group students will often retreat to their own professional group and generalise their experiences, blaming 'the health students' or 'the social workers' for not doing what was expected, replicating experiences from practice.

Applying the public health approach to prevention we can reappraise the family's situation and the analysis of risk to explore the impact of factors as set out by the WHO (2006).

Dr Jones's concerns will focus on the baby's age and her illness. He would also worry about the flat being cold and Mary's apparent lack of responsiveness when he spoke to her. While a social model takes account of all the relevant factors, the medical model is based on consideration of relative risk to the child (see Bungay, Chapter 2 for an explanation of the meanings of relative and absolute risk). Other factors which could indicate risk are the apparent isolation of the young family and their lack of support from parents and the community. Mary's learning disability may also be a contributing factor to concerns about the couples' ability to provide effective parenting for Ebony. However, in weighing up the risk factors it is important not to overlook the rights of the parents (although where these rights conflict with the rights of the child, her needs are paramount (Children Act 2004), and the fact that a social model would suggest that they should if possible be supported to carry out their parental responsibilities rather than these being undermined.

Any mother with a young baby may be tired and unresponsive and the house untidy. When considering risk factors, professional values and anti-discriminatory practice (Thompson 2007) dictate that Mary's learning disability should not be seen in itself as a reason for assuming that she cannot cope.

The current context of practice and resource constraints are likely to lead to greater levels of anxiety and the framing of risk to trigger access to service provision described as 'risk filtration practices' (Hayes and Spratt 2009) whereby 'concerns' are escalated in what are perceived as high risk cases while delegating less dangerous situations to universal service intervention without enforcement. Hayes and Spratt consider that a 'tiered' response to referrals would have a greater impact as the 'threshold' or 'cut off' for child protection intervention does not feed into an evaluative process with any indication of 'near misses', but nevertheless where risk analysis is firmly placed.

Managing the tensions in safeguarding children

There are tensions between health professionals who manage and contain the welfare needs of children within a family but who, when the situation intensifies and with few resources available, may refer the child as in need of protection because the monitoring and surveillance role has indicated this change of circumstance. The role of the health visitor has been considered to be less stigmatising and more welcomed by families (Gimson 2008) than that of the social worker but if the role of the health visitor is to increasingly work with targeted complex families this is likely to cease. Greater surveillance, monitoring and record keeping is intended to allow more efficient access to services, support interprofessional working and enable early intervention, but there is a risk that service users will fail to engage with health services if they feel that they are being monitored and that they cannot trust the professional concerned (Arai 2010).

The importance of supervision and support for those involved in safeguarding

Saunders and Goddard (1998) highlight two key factors which contribute towards good practice in risk assessment as regular and high quality supervision and support, and staff who have the opportunity to evaluate their practice. Reflective practice is at the heart of the health and social care professional in the twenty-first century and it is increasingly recognised that quality clinical supervision for community nurses is important in supporting them to deliver high quality care. Supervision covers the relationship where one worker is given the responsibility to ensure another meets professional and personal objectives as well as certain organisational requirements (Morrison 2001).

Supervision can be varied in quality and purpose and delivered in a variety of ways, to groups, teams or individuals. In health settings the supervisor may be an expert from mental health or a child protection specialist, while in social work settings the predominant model is individual supervision with a line manager or senior colleague. The type of supervision may depend on the needs of the supervisee and/or the availability of supervisors as well as the protocols of the organisation. Child death inquiries have highlighted weaknesses in supervision as a key concern, and even when supervision was being held regularly it was not sufficiently challenging, it was unfocused and superficial and difficult issues were avoided. However, there is concern in health about the generic nature of much of the clinical supervision delivered, for example peer-supervision, which may have little impact on practice while paying lip service to the high profile criticism about the lack of supervision for health visitors (Laming 2003).

Within social work the focus of supervision has shifted to 'management oversight' and ensuring that procedures are followed and that targets have been met, a focus on measurable tasks (Gibbs 2001; Morrison and Wonnacott 2010; Munro 2011).

Child protection supervision requires particular skills; the emotive nature of the work and the anxiety it can engender leads to workers displaying defence mechanisms or displaying an overly punitive attitude towards parents (Munro 2008). As a response to what they may perceive as overly punitive or interfering criticism practitioners may respond by becoming defensive, ignoring instructions or reasserting their power with service users. The supervisor needs skills in challenging and questioning while containing the highly charged emotional aspects of the child protection process (Lister and Crisp 2005).

Practitioners may not always feel safe to reflect openly and honestly on their practice in supervision, particularly if they are supervised by their line manager or if they feel there is a 'blame' culture in their organisation. Historically within nursing and indeed other health professionals the idea of supervision has been held back perhaps due to the workplace culture and stigma attached to signs of poor coping mechanisms as personal weakness. From the supervisees' perspective, time to reflect may be felt to be wasted if it is poorly facilitated, haphazard in its organisation and too infrequent, as well as a misunderstanding that one of the aims of supervision in the helping professionals is restorative (Cutcliffe *et al.* 2001).

Eileen Munro's interim report on child protection has recommended that there should be a greater focus on the emotional and cognitive aspects of supervision, seeing it as a mechanism for helping practitioners to

> critically reflect on the understanding they are forming of the family, of considering their emotional response and whether this is adversely affecting their reasoning, and for making decisions about how best to help. (Munro 2011: 53)

In working with risk this approach provides a basis for challenging bias, acknowledging anxiety and supporting the practitioner in working with the uncertainty which is inherent in the work.

> Firstly, [supervision] must convey the value of individual workers to the children and families they work with and the organization. Secondly, it needs to affirm both the merit and the necessity of exploring the impact of feelings and thoughts on action and perception. Thirdly, it must take more account of adult learning theory and the role of the supervisor in promoting effective learning by workers. (Gibbs 2001)

Conclusions

It can be seen that assessing and managing risk in safeguarding children generates high levels of anxiety and can lead to tensions in interprofessional working due to different conceptualisations of risk and different ideas about who is responsible for managing risk. The concern with making a 'right' decision together with a fear of the possible consequences of a mistake can influence the way in which risk is framed and has led to an increasing reliance on procedures. While *Every Child Matters* (2003) and the Children Act 2004 highlighted that safeguarding children should be a shared responsibility, in reality is there a risk that having collective responsibility could mean that no one agency or practitioner takes responsibility?

It is clear that there is a need to refocus on the broader aspects of risks and rights, sharing responsibilities for identification and prevention of risk across professional groups and ensuring adequate support and supervision of all involved in managing risk.

There is a need for those working within safeguarding to maintain 'respectful inquiry' in interprofessional work – to challenge each other as well as to challenge families. Recent research by the Office of the Children's Commissioner for England (2010) found that a common reason for family hostility towards professionals was that they felt that they had different perceptions of the family's problems and needs, and this led to a defensive attitude on the part of both families and professionals. Families stated that if they did not agree with the professional's assessment they were seen as being 'in denial'. This also happens between practitioners who feel that they cannot speak openly in meetings as they do not want to cause conflict (Munro 2008). It is important that there is open dialogue between practitioners and with families and an acceptance that initial assessments may need to be changed, to acknowledge other views on issues of risk and how families will manage these.

Interprofessional learning can have a key role in enabling greater understanding of each other's roles and responsibilities, although this is not without its challenges and tensions. A shared learning session can be used as a safe environment in which to begin to challenge the assumptions, perceived hierarchies of knowledge and stereotyping that can hinder effective interprofessional communication, although this needs careful facilitation. A shared learning session can enable reflective practice and more creative problem-solving techniques, although research highlights the challenges involved in 'relearning'; lecturers on post-qualifying study programmes are often faced with significant resistance from practitioners to analyse their practice, much of which is intuitive, and potential reluctance to 'unlearn' some behaviours in order to develop their practice further as this can be deskilling and threatening (Mayhew 1999).

Having a shared activity and a shared goal can lead to better integrated working and build up stronger understanding of what each practitioner can contribute to safeguarding (Carpenter and Dickinson 2008). Another key tool for supporting effective interprofessional assessment and management of risk is supervision, as highlighted above. Effective supervision should enable practitioners to manage the uncertainty and anxiety that working with risk can engender. While assessment tools can be useful, there is a risk that over-reliance on procedural tools can lead to an expectation that practitioners will always make the 'right' assessment and ignores the complexity of working with risk (Calder 2008: 50).

It is important to be aware of how different models and perspectives from health and social work can impact on working relationships within the realm of safeguarding, and how this can lead at times to risk-averse practice. However, a shared approach that assesses risk within the wider context of rights and responsibilities can help to promote better understanding of the challenges the work presents for all involved.

References

Allport, G. W. (1954) *The Nature of Prejudice*. Reading, MA: Addison-Wesley.

Appleton, J. V. (1996) Working with vulnerable families: a health visiting perspective. *Journal of Advanced Nursing*, 23(5): 912–18.

Appleton, J. V. and Cowley, S. (2004) The guideline contradiction: health visitors' use of formal guidelines for identifying and assessing families in need. *International Journal of Nursing Studies*, 41: 785–97.

Arai, L. (2010) The surveillance of children young people and families. In L. O'Dell and S. Leverett (eds), *Working with Children and Young People: Co-constructing Practice*. Basingstoke: Palgrave Macmillan.

Ashford, M. and Thomas, J. (2005) Interprofessional education. In H. Burgess and I. Taylor (eds), *Effective Learning and Teaching in Social Policy and Social Work.* Abingdon: Routledge Farmer.

Audit Commission (1994) *Seen but Not Heard: Coordinating Community Health and Social Services for Children in Need.* London: HMSO.

Barber, C., McLaughlin, N. and Wood, J. (2009) Self-awareness: The key to person-centred care? In G. Koubel and H. Bungay (eds), *The Challenge of Person-Centred Care: An Interprofessional Perspective.* Basingstoke: Palgrave Macmillan.

Barker, R. (ed.) (2009) *Making Sense of Every Child Matters: Multi-professional Practice Guidance.* Bristol: Policy Press.

Calder, M. (ed.) (2008) *Contemporary Risk Assessment in Safeguarding Children.* Lyme Regis: Russell House.

Carpenter, J. and Dickinson, H. (2008) *Interprofessional Education and Training.* Bristol: Policy Press.

Corby, B. (2005) *Child Abuse: Towards a Knowledge Base* (3rd edn). Maidenhead: Open University Press.

Cutcliffe, J., Butterworth, T. and Proctor, B. (eds) (2001) *Fundamental Themes in Clinical Supervision.* London: Routledge.

Dalziel, Y. (2008) Community development as a public health function. In S. Cowley (ed.), *Community Public Health in Policy and Practice: A Sourcebook.* London: Baillière Tindall.

Department for Children, Schools and Families (2007) *The Children's Plan: Building Brighter Futures.* London: The Stationery Office.

Department for Education and Skills (2003) *Every Child Matters: Change for Children.* London: DfES.

Department of Health (1991) *Working Together under the Children Act 1989: A Guide to Arrangements for Interagency Co-operation for the Protection of Children from Abuse.* London: HMSO.

Department of Health (1995) *Child Protection: Messages from Research.* London: HMSO.

Department of Health (2002) *Safeguarding Children: A Joint Chief Inspectors' Report on Arrangements to Safeguard Children.* London: Department of Health.

Department of Health (2009) *Healthy Child Programme: The Two Year Review.* London: Department of Health.

Department of Health (2010) *Healthy Child Programme for Pregnancy and the First Five Years of Life.* London: Department of Health.

Gibbs, J. (2001) Maintaining front-line workers in child protection: a case for refocusing supervision. *Child Abuse Review*, 10: 323–35.

Gilbert, R., Spatz, C., Widom, C., Browne, K., Fergusson, D., Webb, E. and Janson, S. (2009) The consequences of child maltreatment in high-income countries. *The Lancet*, 373: 68–81.

Gimson, S. (2008) *Listening to Mother: Making Britain Mother-friendly.* London: Family and Parenting Institute.

Hayes, D. and Spratt, T. (2009) Child welfare interventions: patterns of social work practice. *British Journal of Social Work*, 39: 1575–97.

Holland, S. (2011) *Child and Family Assessment in Social Work Practice.* London: Sage.

Kirton, D. (2009) *Child Social Work: Policy and Practice.* London: Sage.

Laming, Lord (2003) *The Victoria Climbié Inquiry: Report of an Inquiry by Lord Laming.* London: The Stationery Office.

Lister, P. G. and Crisp, B. R. (2005) Clinical supervision in child protection for community nurses. *Child Abuse Review*, 14: 57–72.

Lupton, C., North, N. and Khan, P. (2001) *Working Together or Pulling Apart? The NHS and Child Protection Networks*. Bristol: Policy Press.

Marmot, M. (2010) *Fairer Society Healthier Lives: Strategic Review of Health Inequalities in England Post-2010* (The Marmot Review). London.

Mayhew, J. (1999) Theory, practice and the psychology of expertise. *Social Work Education*, 18(2): 195–206.

Morrison, T. (2001) *Staff Supervision in Social Care: Making a Real Difference for Staff and Service Users*. Brighton: Pavilion Publishing.

Morrison, T. and Wonnacott, J. (2010) *Supervision: Now or Never Reclaiming Reflective Supervision in Social Work*. Available at: http://www.in-trac.co.uk/reclaiming-reflective-supervision.php (accessed 28 March 2011).

Munro, E. (2008) *Effective Child Protection* (2nd edn). London: Sage.

Munro, E. (2011) *The Munro Review of Child Protection Interim Report: The Child's Journey*. Available at: http://www.education.gov.uk/munroreview/firstreport.shtml (accessed 23 March 2011).

Office of the Children's Commissioner for England (2010) *Family perspectives on safeguarding and on relationships with children's services* Available at: http://www.childrenscommissioner.gov.uk/content/publications/content_405 (accessed 24 March 2011).

Parton, N. (ed.) (1997) *Child Protection and Family Support: Tensions, Contradictions and Possibilities*. London: Routledge.

Parton, N. (2006) *Safeguarding Childhood: Early Intervention and Surveillance in a Late Modern Society*. Basingstoke: Palgrave Macmillan.

Parton, N. (2009) From Seebohm to *Think Family*: reflections on 40 years of policy change of statutory children's social work in England. *Child and Family Social Work*, 14: 68–78.

Powell, C. (2007) *Safeguarding Children and Young People: A Guide for Nurses and Midwives*. Maidenhead: Open University Press.

Rose, M. and Killien, M. (1983) Risk and vulnerability: a case for differentiation. *Advances in Nursing Science*, 5(3): 60–73.

Saunders, B. and Goddard, C. (1998) *A Critique of Structured Risk Assessment Procedures: Instruments of Abuse?* Australian Childhood Foundation and the National Research Centre for the Prevention of Child Abuse at Monash University, Melbourne.

Smith, R. (2008) *Social Work with Young People*. Cambridge: Polity Press.

Taylor, C. (2009) Safeguarding children: historical contexts and current landscapes. In K. Broadhurst, C. Grover and J. Jamieson (eds), *Critical Perspectives on Safeguarding Children*. Chichester: Wiley-Blackwell.

Taylor, H., Beckett, C. and McKeigue, B. (2008) Judgements of Solomon: anxieties and defences of social workers involved in care proceedings. *Child and Family Social Work*, 13: 23–31.

Taylor, J. and Daniel, B. (2005) *Child Neglect: Practice Issues for Health and Social Care*. London: Jessica Kingsley.

Thompson, N. (2007) *Power and Empowerment*. Lyme Regis: Russell House.

World Health Organisation (2006) *Preventing Child Maltreatment: A Guide to Taking Action and Generating Evidence*. Geneva: World Health Organisation.

Interprofessional Working and the Community Care Conundrum

Jane Arnott and Georgina Koubel

Introduction

Everyone thinks they know what is meant by community care but the chances are that everybody's understanding of what it means is slightly different. It is often out in the community where practitioners encounter most directly the interface between health and social care, and where the greatest skill is required in order to achieve an acceptable balance between the rights, risks and responsibilities of all the stakeholders involved, whether they are in the receipt or the provision of community care or part of the wider community. Community care has been the watchword for at least a generation of health and welfare policy makers, and as a result there have been significant changes in the ways such services are provided. Issues of interprofessional collaboration have been both challenged and enhanced by the modernisation agenda (Department of Health 1998) to provide 'seamless' services that effectively meet the needs of vulnerable people living in the community.

This chapter explores issues of rights, risks and responsibilities in relation to working with people in community settings. The relationships formed among professionals from diverse professional backgrounds can have a significant impact on the experience for patients and service users living in the community. At times there is lack of clarity about the roles and relationships between, for example, a community care manager and the community matron. Often it is not only the patient or service user who is confused, and this chapter starts by exploring the meanings and significance of community and the roles and responsibilities of the people who are involved in trying to understand the community care conundrum.

Working with people living in the community changes and often complicates the relationships between professionals and service users; the views, perspectives and values of carers, friends and other stakeholders may have significant consequences for the individual who requires health and/or social work or social care services in the community. Particularly in cases where people are perceived as being frail or vulnerable, their choices and wishes to remain in their own homes may depend on the willingness and capacity of what could be called the 'informal care network' of family, friends and neighbours to support the individual to remain in the community as much as the 'formal' or 'professional' support from practitioners within health and social care systems.

This chapter highlights certain dilemmas in relation to the rights of autonomous persons to choose to take risks alongside the issues of the professional responsibility for those who are considered too vulnerable or incapacitated to make decisions for themselves. This may be a particular concern for some older people and their families, for example when working with older people who become increasingly confused or mentally unwell through the progression of dementia. At times there are concerns that families and sometimes professionals can be too quick to assume the role of decision-maker when engaging with older people and people who have disabilities, particularly in areas where there are concerns about risk (Koubel and Bungay 2009). The chapter further considers the requirement for understanding how the power dynamics work in relation to the people involved with someone who may be perceived as frail or vulnerable but who wishes to remain in their own home. Consideration of the role of the practitioner includes analysis of how the power relationships inherent in practice can either inhibit or promote partnership working (S. Thompson 2007) and an understanding of rights and responsibilities in decision making in health and social care.

Policy initiatives may specify nomenclature and highlight certain practices, although they often leave room for interpretation (Johns 2011). Emphasis has rightly been placed on the importance of effective interprofessional working but the perspectives, values and attitudes of practitioners can also lead to a difference in the understanding and application of how individuals manage the balance of rights, risks and responsibilities. In the spirit of improving interprofessional working and a belief in the benefits of developing a critical understanding of alternative perspectives, the chapter looks at a number of complex or contested concepts in health and social care; including:

- community care, care/case management and community matrons

- medical and social models of care and their implications for managing risk

- language/inter-agency working and other role/task descriptors

- perceptions of professional identity and accountability, e.g. 'duty of care'

- exploring ageist attitudes around vulnerability and (in)capacity in practice.

By the end of the chapter you should have developed your understanding of:

- The meanings attached to notions of community and community care

- Individual and groups' sense of community and attitudes around caring responsibilities

- The language and roles attributed to relevant health and social care professionals working with vulnerable people in the community

- The application of the values and diverse perspectives and models of different professionals working with vulnerable adults living within the community

- The legal and ethical challenges involved in maintaining vulnerable people in the community, taking into account rights, mental capacity, choice and safety

- The dilemmas and conflicts that arise in balancing rights, risks and responsibilities when working with individuals who may be vulnerable, their carers and the wider community.

The chapter draws on case studies and reflective exercises in the form of challenges to provide opportunities to explore the application of the principles of social capital, and to develop awareness of the practice dilemmas involved in working with older people and other vulnerable people in the community. The objective is to enable reflection on personal and professional values and critical practice analysis.

The introduction of community care and care management into the health and welfare systems in the United Kingdom had a profound impact on the balance of rights, risks and responsibilities. The principles envisioned in the Barclay Report (1982), *The Social Basis of Community Care*, and in *Caring for People: Community Care in the Next Decade and Beyond* (Department of Health 1989) was enshrined in a key piece of legislation, the National Health Service and Community Care Act 1990. Those who were the intended recipients of the changes, that is, 'those who may need community care services' were largely those people considered to be among the most vulnerable in society. This legislation also introduced the concept of care management into health and welfare provision for older people, for people with long-term conditions, learning and/or physical disabilities and for people with mental health difficulties.

Blakemore (2003) provides a good general introduction to the social policy changes that heralded de-institutionalisation of people with mental health difficulties and disabilities and provides a useful analysis of the impact of community care reforms in both health and social care. The significance of the introduction of community care and the Care Programme Approach (the mental health equivalent of care management) within both social care and mental health services has been critically explored by Hadley and Clough (1996). However, this chapter will concentrate on looking at the ways in which issues of rights, risks and responsibilities affect older people and people with disabilities living in the community.

What do we mean by 'community care'?

The introduction of community care has raised many issues about professional and interprofessional roles and the allocation of resources. This has led to further policy developments which have had a significant impact on people who use health and social care services (Johns 2011). Before exploring these in more detail, it is helpful to start by looking at the meanings of the terms 'community', 'community care' and 'care management' and the implications of these ways of working for practice in health and social care.

CHALLENGE

■ What does the term 'community' mean to you?

■ What 'communities' are important to you?

The term 'community' is a highly contested concept as it involves a complex interplay of different meanings and perspectives (Arnott 2010). Community is considered to be of significant value as it contributes positively to the well-being of society as a whole and as Robson (2000) asserts, is seen to support notions of cooperation, cohesion and inclusivity, which are essential components of a civilised society.

Cohen (1985) contends that communities are born out of a sense of commonality:

■ place communities describe a shared place of residence;

■ interest communities describe shared characteristics such as ethnic origin or occupation;

■ communities of attachment describe a shared agreement which brings people together.

These terms are not necessarily mutually exclusive to one another and invariably overlap, for example a religious community could be described as a group of individuals who may share a religious belief (interest) and worship in the same church (place) – Crow and Allen (1995).

One of the criticisms of communities of place is that they are often defined by outsiders or governmental organisations, either for ease of administration or to delineate one geographical community from another. In effect, the defined community may have more meaning for those defining the geographical boundaries, than the residents themselves. Commonality of place does not necessarily mean that individuals will have much to do with each other, furthermore disadvantaged groups of the marginalised and powerless are more likely to be missed when definitions of community defined by an outsider are applied (Jewkes and Murcott 1996).

More recent research into the meaning of community indicates that it is the social networks and relationships which give us our sense of community. Putnam (2000) suggests that these factors not only give us our sense of self and individuality but also empower us to manage the strains and stresses of modern day living. White (2009) asserts that consideration must always be given to the quality of networks and relationships in the development of any care package as this knowledge can positively affect the outcome of such activity. It also alerts us to the risks and helps to identify where duty and responsibilities lie.

Social capital describes how networks and shared norms promote community cooperation, mutual benefit and civic engagement (Putnam 2000). There is a clear relationship between the quality of social capital and the health experience of the population. Poor social capital which arises from poverty or social marginalisation has a direct link with reduced health, whereas high social capital has been identified as a protective factor against poor health (De Silva *et al.* 2005). The key factors which provide this protection appear to be a level of mutual trust and cooperation.

CASE STUDY: SOCIAL CAPITAL, CHOICE AND THE ROLE OF THE STATE

Philip and Colin are brothers and continue to live in their childhood home, which was recently left to them after the death of their mother. Philip has learning difficulties and now relies on Colin for support in his day-to-day care. Colin retired from his job at a local supermarket after his mother died to look after his brother, who is in his early seventies. Colin is 65 years old.

Philip requires help with washing and dressing, and supervision when he is preparing food and drink. Colin tries very hard to maintain a routine, as Philip becomes stressed when the routine changes. Colin can only leave Philip for very short periods of time as Philip also has a tendency to wander. The local community support officer (CSO) knows the brothers well and has found Philip wandering and brought him home on several occasions. The CSO visits occasionally and Colin appreciates these visits as it helps him connect with the outside world.

The social worker who has known the family for years became increasingly concerned for both brothers after the death of their mother. Colin became depressed after losing his mother and retiring from his job. Colin is adamant that he will continue to look after his brother. He has lots of interests but has had to give some of these up to care for Philip. The brothers have supportive neighbours and friends who help with shopping and transport and sit with Philip when Colin has to go out. Colin feels reluctant to ask for extra help as he feels ultimately responsible for Philip.

================= **CHALLENGE** =================

■ What do you think are the brothers' needs?

■ What do you think might be done to meet these needs?

| **CASE STUDY continued** |

The social worker knows that Colin has always wanted to own an allotment and suggested that they might like to get involved in a local allotment group which aims to promote the health and well-being of individuals. She explains that the way the group has been set up would be appropriate for both brothers. After some consideration, Colin and Philip join the Allotment Group.

The members of the Allotment Group are very friendly and inclusive and in a very short time, Colin feels comfortable enough to allow Philip to go to the allotment on occasions by himself. Members of the group come to the house to collect Philip at a specified time of day, so that Colin has some time to enjoy his other interests and meet up with old friends.

Colin appears less depressed and is delighted with the improvement in his brother. He believes the exercise and social contact has made the brothers fitter and happier. He recently told the social worker that he realised he could not do everything for Philip and that the Allotment Group had provided a safety valve for what was becoming a very stressful situation.

================= **CHALLENGE** =================

■ What do you feel about the social worker's intervention?

■ How does the referral to the Allotment Group meet the needs of the brothers?

■ How does it demonstrate respect for Colin's and Philip's beliefs and values?

The outcome for Philip and Colin at this point appears to be a positive one. It is also a good example of how important it is for professionals to understand the needs of individuals and families and to consider and respect the beliefs and values of individuals as care plans are developed. Colin's sense of responsibility for his brother is very strong and involves a range of caring activities, some of which might be considered to be very intimate and inappropriate for a brother to undertake. It would be possible to obtain assistance from an appropriate agency but Colin feels that although he finds this difficult, he should continue as his mother used to provide personal care for Philip and this is what Philip has become accustomed to.

CHALLENGE

■ What do you think of Colin's expectations of himself?

■ Do you think it would be better for Philip's personal care to be taken on by an external agency or that it should continue to be provided by his brother?

■ What factors influence your viewpoint?

One solution might be to fund a carer from social services to undertake some of the day-to-day caring responsibilities and ease the stress for Colin. However, in theory at least, contemporary health and social care provision is underpinned by concepts such as community care, maintaining independence, empowerment, social inclusion and respect for diversity as well as care and protection for vulnerable people (Waine *et al.* 2005). The social worker understands this and demonstrates respect for Colin and Philip's wishes and would not wish to undermine Colin's belief that he is the best person to care for his brother. However, Colin acknowledges that he finds it stressful and the risk in this situation is that he may feel overwhelmed and unable to carry on the caring role if it becomes too much for him. One way of maintaining Colin's caring role, and potentially of promoting Philip's independence in the longer term, would be to support Colin in undertaking those aspects of Philip's care that he finds acceptable and see if it is possible to arrange for someone else to take on the roles he finds more difficult. The involvement of an external agency could also provide a useful monitoring role to help the brothers manage in their changed circumstances.

In addition to the input of social services, the referral to the Allotment Group provides a support mechanism that promotes independence, empowerment and social inclusion. The social worker does not ignore the risk factors in Colin and Philip's case, but is able to balance these against the context of where they live, the acceptance and quality of support from neighbours and friends and Colin and Philip's coping strategies. Another way of describing what the social worker understands is the protective role that social capital can afford individuals when managing difficult situations (Putnam 2000). Her suggestion of the Allotment Group aims to strengthen this protective role as well as accepting the brothers' wants and desires and treating them with dignity and respect. Instead of either 'taking over' the care of Philip or leaving Colin to cope on his own, this plan enables risks to be managed through a combination of state intervention, family responsibility and social capital.

Perspectives on community care and care management

The idea of people being cared for in the community, by the community or on behalf of the community goes back throughout history and relates to all times and all places but the ways in which this is understood by society and the ways in which help, support, care etc. are provided depends on the political and ideological context. Community care and care management have been corner-stones of service provision within the UK over the past 20 years at least but there can be some confusion about what any of these terms really mean within the context of health and social care. It is helpful therefore to start this section with some reflection on terms which are commonly used but not always clearly understood.

In social work and social care, the title 'care manager' or 'case manager' (originating in the United States) can almost be seen as interchangeable. The name carries no formal status, as would be required from someone who called themselves a nurse, an occupational therapist or a social worker, but a care manager can be any of these, or they may have no formal professional qualifications. Care managers have no overarching governing body, while nurses, social workers and occupational therapists, all of whom may be employed in the care management role, are required to register with their own registering bodies. The term 'case manager' has replaced care manager in some areas as it is felt to be more appropriate for people who are accessing individual budgets as part of the personalisation agenda, where the relationship is perceived to be more about managing the 'case' of the person who is enabled to access their own support services rather than commissioning and managing their care for them.

Personalisation is yet another method of managing services to people in the community, usually older people or people with disabilities where people are allocated individual budgets under the Direct Payments Act 2006 to purchase their own choice of care. Although not restricted to social work, personalisation is seen as the first choice for people wishing to access community care services. Because it offers the opportunity for service users to manage their own finances under the Direct Payments Act 2006, it is seen as generally a positive and empowering process whereby people who need to access services achieve a greater degree of control over how the finances they are allotted by the local authority can be spent (Gardner 2011). This links with the assumption that most people given the choice would prefer to take on responsibility for managing their services themselves. However, for some more vulnerable members of the community this may also raise issues of potential tensions between the service user's assessment of their needs and the views of the care/case manager. There is also a potential conflict between the rights of the service user and the management of risks as a result of practitioners playing a reduced role in the monitoring and review of the services provided (Gardner 2011).

For many people the opportunity to manage their own money and purchase services of their choice can be a very positive experience while for others it may be less so, particularly if they have limited experience or preparation for the process of undertaking the responsibilities involved. It certainly highlights many of the concerns that have been discussed throughout this book about the difficulties of balancing rights, risks and responsibilities (SCIE 2010) for vulnerable people living in the community.

At its simplest level, community care refers to people living in the community rather than in institutions. There is in fact no agreed definition of community care (Johns 2011) but whatever terms or methods are used, every community has to find ways of promoting the health and well-being of its more vulnerable members (Brown 2010). As we no longer agree that it is generally acceptable, except in extreme circumstances where people are a risk to themselves or others, to keep people with disabilities and people with mental health problems locked up in asylums (Mental Health Act 1983), care in the community is an inevitable part of the factors that have to be considered when we think about how we as individuals and as societies react and respond to people with a wide array of different needs.

Commentators such as Carr (2001) describe community as a broad landscape where the impact of the determinants of health and social well-being is more visible and needs to be considered as part of any care plan. Community nursing has a long tradition – Florence Nightingale wrote extensively throughout her life about community nursing and recognised the importance and difference of approach of nursing in this context.

> Never think you have done anything effectual in nursing in London, til you nurse, not only the sick poor in workhouses, but those at home. (Florence Nightingale 1867, cited in Monteiro 1985: 1).

Most importantly, Florence Nightingale recognised the importance of understanding the link between poverty, environment, lifestyle and disease and was a staunch advocate of incorporating this into community nursing education. Nightingale believed that the nurses' role apart from nursing the sick was to teach the poor about cleanliness and sanitation in an attempt to reduce infectious disease. Attitudes and the paternalistic approach have changed significantly since the introduction of community nursing; community nurses continue to be the main providers of professional nursing care in the patient's home and adopt a collaborative approach to care (Nursing Midwifery Council 2008). Peter (2002) describes the relationship between nurse and individual, family and community as one where a working partnership approach is essential and where the respect for the wants, desires and negotiated solutions to needs, are worked through.

The National Health Service has undergone significant change within the last few years. This has been driven by a modernising agenda which has reviewed roles and services and sought ways to bring care closer to home (Sines *et al.* 2009).

As a result of this need for change, new roles have emerged in order for individuals to work across organisations to reduce costs, improve quality of care and streamline services. The process of service integration is complex as the philosophy, values and culture of these different organisations can at times appear to be at odds with one another. Haynes (2003) argues that organisations need to move away from a silo mentality, towards one that recognises the need for organisational co-dependency, where boundaries become soft and permeable

and clarity and transparency are promoted. This not only benefits the organisations but supports individuals, families and communities, as they navigate their
way through complex bureaucratic systems in order to meet their health and
social care needs.

Sines *et al.* (2009) argue that community nurses have always been at the
interface between health and social care organisations as they assess need and
plan care; indeed the ability to network is an essential community nursing skill.
However, the roles and responsibilities of the community nurse have had to
change, in order to meet the growing health and social needs of an ever-increas-
ing ageing population who will be living with long-term conditions such as
diabetes, cardiac failure and dementia (Murphy 2004).

Social work, care managers, case managers and community matrons

Social work, although originating from the philanthropists and political ideal-
ists of the nineteenth century, as a profession can be traced back to the early
twentieth century when the trials and hardships experienced by the poor and
those afflicted by age and mental and physical disability was recognised as a
legitimate concern of the state. The role grew throughout the latter part of the
twentieth century until the ideology of universal services was challenged by the
Conservative Government of 1979 who wanted to limit the involvement of the
state in relation to vulnerable groups and individuals, partly on grounds of cost
and partly because of the fear of creating welfare dependency (see Adams,
Chapter 3 for further discussion about the change in ideology). Care management as a method of social work was introduced by the NHS and Community
Care Act.

It was seen ideologically as a way both to address standards of care and to
reduce the expenditure and the responsibility of the state in health and social
care for vulnerable people (Means and Smith 1998: 45). The best way of
achieving this, it was felt, was to separate the commissioning of services from
those who provided them, therefore bringing into the welfare system the
concept of the marketplace as regulator of 'community care services'.

The modernisation of health and social care services has led to the requirement for health and welfare practitioners to work more closely together to
provide a 'seamless service' (Department of Health 1998) to more vulnerable
people in the community who are suffering from more complicated long-term
conditions. One government initiative to meet these challenges has been the
introduction of the community matron (Department of Health 2004, 2005).
Community matrons proactively 'case manage' individuals with highly complex
needs, and possess advanced knowledge, skills and experience to work as the
case manager; coordinating care between an individual's GP, hospital and other
agencies such as social services. The patient's interests, desires and wants are key
to the development of personalised care plans in order to prevent deterioration

of an individual's condition and where possible, to prevent unplanned admission to hospital (Murphy 2004).

Case management involves the care of individuals who are the main users of unplanned secondary care. As the model of care shows, this high risk group of patients needs not only good management of their specific diseases, but also a holistic overview to be taken of their full health and social care needs. Their care should go beyond the clinical to encompass the full range of factors that affect them, such as their ability to maintain personal interests and social contact.

The success of this initiative is dependent upon several factors which include inter-agency collaboration in case management planning and clarity of the community matron role. Research from the King's Fund (Goodwin *et al.* 2010), however, has identified that there is a range of interpretations of the term 'case management', with some viewing it as a team process rather than one person's role. There is further confusion as now some care managers have been designated as case managers but they do not carry out the role of community matrons, and vice versa. Whoever carries it out, case management is a difficult role and its complexity underestimated. This difference in perception may pose a risk for the individual undertaking the role, as other colleagues may not be clear about the community matron's responsibilities, skills and expertise, and how these interact with those of a social worker or nurse who is also called a case manager but who works for social services and whose role may be very different. This will be a matter for interprofessional negotiation to ensure roles and responsibilities are clearly understood (Quinney 2006).

In social work, care management has for the past twenty years, at least until recently, been the primary method and model for working with 'people who need community care services'. Previously those people who worked for social services with older people and people with disabilities had generally been social workers, some of whom may have specialised in practice in this area, or social workers who had been working in a generic way with a range of people such as children and families, people with mental health difficulties etc., including some older and disabled people on their caseloads.

The development of community care highlighted the role of social work ethics and values and the sometimes conflicting and contradictory nature of their accountabilities (Banks 2006). These tensions might mean that in a complex situation involving one or more service users, their families, the community, social expectations (of, for example, older people or of professional practitioners), by agencies and by the media may conflict with the values of the practitioners or there may be a clash of values and perspectives between practitioners and among any of the other parties. While conflict can be constructed as potentially positive and creative (Quinney 2006) it is more likely, particularly in cases involving rights, risks and responsibilities that these conflicts will potentially aggravate and be aggravated by the different views and agendas involved. Think carefully about issues to do with our attitudes towards older people in our society, then have a look at the following case study and then take time to reflect on the questions that follow.

━━━━━━━━━━━━━━━━━ **CHALLENGE** ━━━━━━━━━━━━━━━━━

Age, vulnerability and autonomy in older people

■ What images come to your mind when you think about 'older people' or 'the elderly'?

■ Where do you think your ideas come from?

■ How do you think they could affect the way you would work with older people?

'Older people' is a very wide construct. It is difficult even to start to think about at what age, age becomes an issue. Some people who are chronologically old appear in some ways much younger than their peers, while we all know people who seem to hit middle age before they are even out of their teens. You may be one of many people who either think that you have a positive and proactive approach to older age, or ageism may be something that you assume you and possibly other people have never personally encountered – yet. However, the beliefs we have been brought up with about older people, whether it is a matter of respecting our elders, being aware of the burden of an ageing population, or assuming that old people need, or even deserve protection because they are inevitably frailer and more vulnerable than the rest of us, all affect the way we are likely to engage and work with older people.

━━━━━━━━━━━━━━━━━ **CHALLENGE** ━━━━━━━━━━━━━━━━━

'Increasingly, as people grow older, one of the pervading experiences faced is that of ageism' (Phillips *et al.* 2006: 46).

■ What do you think ageism actually is? Look at the elements in the list below.

■ What do you think is meant by each of the concepts included in the following list, and how do you think such attitudes may affect the experiences and the rights of older people within society?

■ What do you understand by each of these words? How do they relate to older people and people with disabilities? What is the significance for this in terms of peoples' rights?

☐ Infantilisation (patronising or talking down to someone as if to a child or a baby)
☐ Medicalisation (dealing with problems by giving medication only)
☐ Marginalisation (not including people in mainstream services)
☐ Dehumanisation (not thinking of the person as fully human as oneself)
☐ Internalisation of oppression (the person accepting stereotyped views of self)
☐ Denial of citizenship rights (assuming some people cannot participate in society)
☐ Life course expectations (making assumptions about people's wishes and needs based on their age alone, or equating age or disability only with negative characteristics).

CASE STUDY

Mrs Gold is a widow in her eighties living alone in a second floor privately rented flat in a large converted house. The other tenants in the house are mainly much younger than Mrs Gold and in general keep themselves pretty much to themselves. This suits Mrs Gold as she is very independent and hates to ask anyone for help. She is normally quite smartly dressed and goes out to the shops and the library and worked as a volunteer cook at the local luncheon club a couple of times a week. Recently Mrs Gold spent several weeks in hospital following a fall which led to a broken ankle, fractured wrist and severe bruising along her side. She lay for several hours before a neighbour alerted the ambulance service and Mrs Gold was almost hypothermic by the time she was admitted to hospital. When discharge was discussed, Mrs Gold told the hospital staff that she has a daughter, Sarah, who calls in on a regular basis to see her mother and help out with shopping, cooking and housework. In general this level of contact had enabled Mrs Gold to maintain her independence in the community, and hospital staff decided that as there was a daughter nearby no referral to social services was necessary.

Mrs Gold values her relationship with her daughter and has always felt it is important to her that she and Sarah have an amicable and equitable relationship. Sarah phones most evenings but as she works full time and lives several miles away, she only visits her mother two or three times a month. However, on her most recent visit which she made a week or so after Mrs Gold's discharge from hospital, Sarah found her mother appeared distant and unresponsive and looked as if she had lost weight. Her clothes were unkempt, and she hardly spoke to her, except to say she was fine and didn't need any help. Community nurses say that the ankle is mending quite well but they fear that Mrs Gold may be getting depressed as she finds it so difficult to go out and meet with her friends. Other residents in Mrs Gold's building have told you that they think Mrs Gold is not eating and appears dirty and neglected. They think Sarah should take her mother to live with her as Mrs Gold 'obviously cannot look after herself any longer'. Sarah does not want to force her mother to live with her but she feels she will be neglecting her if she leaves her alone in her current situation.

CHALLENGE

- What are the risks in this situation?
- Who has what rights?
- What personal and professional responsibilities are relevant here?
- How could the attitudes and values of the parties involved affect the situation?

The temptation is to look at this case scenario primarily in terms of the risks involved. Mrs Gold is certainly chronologically among the group whom others would identify as 'older people' although that does not mean that she sees herself in this way (Stuart-Hamilton 2006). She has been independent and autonomous until this current crisis and may have difficulty in perceiving herself as being 'at risk', although other residents who have a paternalistic or ageist approach to the needs of older people may well feel they are suggesting what is best for her. Thinking about the list of words and qualities that inform ageism, there is a considerable risk that those around her will take a paternalistic approach which will further affect Mrs Gold's self-esteem and self-respect and which could contribute to loss of independence and her sense of autonomy. One way to address these risks (as well as those that other people are expressing concerns about) will be to ensure that any risk assessments and any resulting decisions are carried out with Mrs Gold at the centre of the process.

Carson and Bain (2008, cited in Galpin and Bates 2009: 24) suggest risk assessment involves two variable factors – outcomes and likelihood. Mrs Gold may or may not want her daughter to be involved in a process of risk assessment. In this situation, it is the responsibility of the practitioner to spell out potential risks and identify the rights, choices and options that are open to Mrs Gold. In this way it should be possible to manage the risks in such a way that Mrs Gold's independence and autonomy is not diminished by the imposition of well-meaning help from other residents or care providers. On the other hand, Mrs Gold has experienced a considerable blow to her sense of herself and her identity as a self-governing, perfectly able individual with position and status in the community. This loss of confidence, or sense of self, may be one of the factors affecting Mrs Gold's ability to recover emotionally or psychologically from the fall as quickly as her physical recovery would indicate.

Rather than trying to avoid risk, it would be better to acknowledge that for older people, as with everyone else, living with risk is a normal part of everyday life (Bornat and Blytheway 2010) and that the involvement of the older person is critical. One way of understanding the significance of the fall for Mrs Gold is to establish a relationship with her, involving her fully in the assessment process, including the assessment and management of any risks involved in her remaining in her own home, if this is what she prefers. In this way, we find out about Mrs Gold the person, explore what is important to her, what she likes and dislikes and whether there are any religious or cultural issues we should be taking into account. We keep Mrs Gold at the centre of any plans and decisions that need to be made and, most importantly, we see her as a person first and patient or a user of services second.

Practitioners may – indeed must – be aware of Mrs Gold's age and her vulnerability, and will certainly have a number of theories and models about people who are that age or who have those areas of vulnerability. A medical model approach would certainly pick up on the fact that Mrs Gold is not eating well and is therefore at risk of malnutrition, and perhaps look to social services to provide Meals on Wheels services. However, this could be seen as a stereotypical response, based on what has normally been supplied to people of a certain age. If we think about Mrs Gold as a person, we should be aware, for example, of issues of loss (Currer 2007) but in applying this approach we need to have listened to the fact that Mrs Gold's loss of status within her local community as a result of the fall may be affecting her ability to re-engage with her peer group. Finding ways to boost her sense of self-worth are essential if Mrs Gold is to avoid slipping into a dependency role that could reduce her quality of life and ultimately increase the financial pressure on health and welfare budgets. The risks of social isolation and loss of status may be far more important to Mrs Gold than her nutritional intake but social interaction may also stimulate her self-esteem, increase her activity levels and therefore improve her appetite.

Rights

In terms of leaving her home and going to live with her daughter, Mrs Gold has an absolute right to refuse to leave her home; whatever risks other people are expressing, she has the human right to make her own decisions unless it can be proved categorically that she does not have the capacity to do so (Human Rights Act 1998; Mental Capacity Act 2005). Not only would it be legally wrong to insist on her moving, the responsibilities of all the stakeholders should be to promote Mrs Gold's rights and maintain Mrs Gold's independence rather than seeking solutions that will undermine it.

It is not unusual for other people to make assumptions about the needs of older people, and to take steps to remove any areas of risk or danger from the lives of older people. Depending on the cultural context of the particular family and their beliefs, this may be either out of respect for the individual or because they feel they are less capable than younger people (Stuart-Hamilton 2006). However, the basic principles of the Human Rights Act apply to Mrs Gold in the same way as everyone else.

1. Right not to be deprived of liberty except in specified circumstances and only in accordance with legal procedure (Article 5)

2. Right to respect for one's home, private and family life (Article 8)

3. Right not to suffer discrimination (Article 14).

These rights clearly establish the fact that Mrs Gold cannot be removed from her home without her consent. The considerable blow accorded to her dignity and self-respect by the fall and the resultant experience of helplessness has probably been exacerbated by the level of concern expressed by others. The risk in this situation is that Mrs Gold will lose her sense of autonomy and start to think it is right that people should start to make decisions for her. It is very important, therefore, that any intervention supports Mrs Gold's dignity and self-respect as these are fundamental to human rights and human relationships.

Conflicting rights and responsibilities

The Mental Capacity Act 2005 states clearly there should be an assumption of capacity unless it can be proven to the contrary. There is no evidence from the above scenario that Mrs Gold has lost her ability to think, reason, understand options or make decisions. There is, however, enough within it to raise issues for others about her ability to cope independently. However, unless there is clear evidence that she is unable to make decisions for herself, she has an absolute right to make up her own mind about what she wants to do, including the right to make 'unwise decisions' if that is her preference. There may well be some tension between what Mrs Gold wants for herself and what other people think would be too risky for her (Orme 2001) but practitioners have a clear commitment to support the rights of the individuals with whom they work and at times may find that their role involves having to make the arguments to support the choices and decisions that older people, and others who may be considered vulnerable, wish to make about remaining in the community (O'Hagan, 2007:233).

Mrs Gold is clearly a capable woman who has recently had a severe blow to her confidence and ability. Setting up a case conference involving all the key stakeholders could reveal significant details about Mrs Gold's situation that may help to find solutions to seemingly intractable problems. For example, in this case it came to light that no one had actually spoken with Mrs Gold about *why* she fell. Despite the policy requirements of the *National Service Framework for Older People* (Department of Health 2001) there was an assumption that she had fallen 'just because of her age'. In fact, under sensitive questioning from the community nurses, Mrs Gold revealed she had fallen because, having to go to the bathroom in the night, an increasingly common occurrence that Mrs Gold herself had thought was due to old age, she had felt dizzy and missed her step. This led to further investigations and once medication was arranged for diabetes she began to feel much better and less anxious about falling again. Realising that her input could significantly affect the decisions that need to be made, Mrs Gold then admitted that she had difficulty using the shower because of her fear of falling again and had told her friends to stay away because she couldn't bear for them to see her in such a state. Some minor adaptations were provided to support her in the shower. By reminding her of her responsibility to participate in keeping safe and allaying the fears of others, her daughter agreed to help Mrs Gold with her hair if she could in return persuade Mrs Gold to wear a Lifeline at night so she could contact someone if she did fall again. As a result, Mrs Gold then felt able to see her friends again and allow them to visit her.

These measures improved Mrs Gold's health and her mental well-being considerably as she took back control of her health and her diet and mood improved. Talking with Mrs Gold about the risks inherent in her situation but keeping in mind both her rights and responsibilities, and the limits of the responsibilities of others, draws on the person-centred attitudes and values that health and social work practitioners sign up to in their codes of conduct and *working with* her rather than *doing to* her not only respects her rights but promotes choice and empowerment (see N. Thompson 2007) in a way that is most likely to maintain Mrs Gold's independence for as long as possible. She recognised that she may need to accept some help for the time being in order to manage to remain in her own home, and there may be some risks involved in the process, but any assistance needs to be provided in a way that will restore confidence and maintain her dignity and self-esteem.

In this case, there are a number of decisions that need to be made, and these need to be addressed in an ethical as well as a systematic way (Bowles *et al.* 2011). Involving Mrs Gold and (with her agreement) other stakeholders like her daughter and possibly other residents in the house, in weighing up carefully the pros and cons of each possible outcome enable the balance of risks, rights and responsibilities to be addressed (Titterton 2005) in order to find the most acceptable solution to the highlighted worries and concerns. Taking a rights-based, interprofessional approach, which shares the responsibility with Mrs Gold (and other relevant stakeholders), led to the formation of a plan that involved the whole system in managing the risk without reducing Mrs Gold's autonomy or denying her choices. Thinking about her as a whole person rather than a stereotype ensured that within the decisions reached, Mrs Gold's rights, wishes and best interests were placed at the heart of the decision-making process, even if in some cases there will always be areas of risk that cannot be fully controlled and the risks have to be balanced against potential gains (Taylor 2010).

Conclusion: risk, rights and choice

To return to the learning outcomes for this chapter, it should be clear that issues that relate to community, care management and community care are not fixed or rigid but liable to change over time. Ideology affects policy and policy affects practice in both health and social care. The way in which policies affect the balance of rights, risks and responsibilities is significant in determining the experience of the outcome for people who may be old, frail and/or otherwise seen to be vulnerable. It is important that risks and concerns are acknowledged but it must also be understood that people in the community have rights and responsibilities, and many people living in the community also have considerable strengths and resilience which they have built up over years of managing the challenges and problems they have dealt with in their lives.

Effective interprofessional working in health and social care requires a good understanding of the perspectives of practitioners from diverse professional backgrounds, and, as in the acute sector, there are times when different perspectives require discussion and resolution to assess and manage the risks. This must be achieved in a way that does not reduce the autonomy or negate the rights and responsibilities of individuals at the heart of practice.

Useful further resources

Community Care – **www.community-care.org.uk**

Social Care Institute of Excellence – **www.scie.org.uk**

Further reading

Alaszeweski, A., Alaszeweski, H., Ayer, S. and Manthorpe, G. (2006) *Managing Risk in Community Practice: Nursing, Risk and Decision Making*. London: Ballière Tindall.

Alcock, E., Daly, C. and Griggs, G. (2008) *Introducing Social Policy* (2nd edn). Harlow: Pearson Educational Graham.

Cattell, V. (2001) Poor people, poor places, and poor health: the mediating role of social networks and social capital. *Social Science and Medicine*, 52(10): 1501–16.

Commission for Social Care Inspection (2008) *Safeguarding Adults: A Study of the Effectiveness of Arrangements to Safeguard Adults from Abuse*. London: CSCI. Available at: http://www.cqc.org.uk/_db/_documents/safeguard[1].pdf

Department of Health (2010) *A Vision for Social Care: Capable Communities and Active Citizens*. London: Department of Health.

Hardy, S. (2009) *Dignity in Health Care for People with Learning Disabilities*. RCN Guidance. London: Royal College of Nursing.

Hutt, R., Rosen, R. and McCaulay, J. (2004) *Review of Literature on the Impact of Case Management on Use of Health Services, Functional Ability and Cost*. London: King's Fund.

Kemshall, H. (1996) *Risk, Social Policy and Welfare*. Buckingham: Open University Press.

Kelly, A. and Symonds, A. (2003) *The Social Construction of Community Nursing*. Basingstoke: Palgrave Macmillan.

Lymbery, M. (2005) *Social Work with Older People: Context, Policy and Practice*. London: Sage.

Malin, N., Wilmot, S. and Manthorpe, J. (2002) *Key Concepts and Debates in Health and Social Policy*. Buckingham: Open University Press.

Mandelstam, M. (2008) *Community Care Practice and the Law* (4th edn) London: Jessica Kingsley.

Mantell, A. (ed.) (2009) *Social Work Skills with Adults*. Exeter: Learning Matters.

Payne, G. (2006) *Social Divisions*. Basingstoke: Palgrave Macmillan.

Purdy, S. (2010) *Avoiding Hospital Admissions: What the Research Evidence Says?* London: The King's Fund.

Webb, S. A. (2006) *Social Work in a Risk Society: Social and Political Perspectives*. Basingstoke: Palgrave Macmillan.

Wellman, B. (2000) Physical place and cyber-place: the rise of networked individualism, *International Journal for Urban and Regional Research*, 25(2): 227–52.

Wolfensberger, W. (1972) *The Principle of Normalization in Human Service*. Toronto: National Institute of Retardation.

References

Arnott, J. (2010) Liberating new talents: an innovative pre-registration community-focused adult nursing programme. *British Journal of Community Nursing*, 15(11): 561–5.

Banks, N. (2006) *Values and Ethics in Social Work* (3rd edn). Basingstoke: Palgrave Macmillan.

Blakemore, K. (2003) *Social Policy: An Introduction* (2nd edn). Buckingham: Open University Press.

Bornat, J. and Blytheway, B. J. (2010) Perceptions and presentations of living with risk in later life. *British Journal of Social Work*, 40(4): 1118–34.

Bowles, W., Collingridge, M., Curry, S. and Valentine, B. (2011) *Ethical Practice in Social Work*. Berkshire: Open University Press/McGraw Hill.

Brown, K. (2010) *Vulnerable Adults and Community Care* (2nd edn). Exeter: Learning Matters.

Carr, S. (2001) Nursing in the community-impact of context on the practice agenda *Journal of Clinical Nursing*, 10(3): 330–6.

Cohen, A. P. (1985) *The Symbolic Construction of Community*. London: Routledge.

Crow, G. and Allan, G. (1994) *Community Life: An Introduction to Local Social Relations*. Hemel Hempstead: Harvester Wheatsheaf.

Currer, C. (2007) *Loss and Social Work*. Exeter: Learning Matters.

Department of Health (1989) *Caring for People: Community Care in the Next Decade and Beyond*. London: HMSO.

Department of Health (1998) *Modernising Social Services*. London: Department of Health.

Department of Health (2001) *National Service Framework for Older People* London: HMSO.

Department of Health (2004) *The NHS Improvement Plan*. London: The Stationery Office.

Department of Health (2005) *Supporting People with Long term Conditions: An NHS and Social Care Model to Support Local Innovation and Integration*. London: The Stationery Office.

De Silva, M., McKenzie, K., Harpham, T. and Huttly, S. (2005) Social capital and mental illness: a systematic review. *Journal of Epidemiology and Community Health*, 59: 619–27.

Galpin, D. and Bates, N. (2009) *Social Work Practice with Adults*. Exeter: Learning Matters.

Gardner, A. (2011) *Personalisation in Social Work*. Exeter: Learning Matters.

Goodwin, N., Curry, N., Naylor, C., Ross, S. and Duldig, W. (2010) *Managing People with Long Term Conditions*, Research paper. London: King's Fund.

Hadley, R. and Clough, I. (1996) *Care in Chaos: Frustration and Challenge in Community Care*. London: Cassell.

Haynes, P. (2003) *Managing Complexity in the Public Services*. Maidenhead: Open University Press.

Jewkes, R. and Murcott, A. (1996) Meanings of community. *Social Science and Medicine*, 43: 555–63.

Johns, R. (2011) *Social Work, Social Policy and Older People*. Exeter: Learning Matters.

Koubel, G. and Bungay, H. (2009) *The Challenge of Person-Centred Care: An Interprofessional Perspective*. Basingstoke: Palgrave Macmillan.

Means, R. and Smith, R. (1998) *Community Care: Policy and Practice* (2nd edn). Hampshire: Palgrave Macmillan.

Monteiro, L. (1985) Public health then and now: Florence Nightingale on public health nursing. *American Journal of Public Health*, 75(2): 181–6.

Murphy, E. (2004) Case management and community matrons for long term condition: a tough job that will need highly trained professionals. *British Medical Journal*, 329(7477): 1251–2.

Nursing Midwifery Council (2008) *Standards of Conduct, Performance and Ethics for Nurses and Midwives.* London: NMC.

O'Hagan, K. (ed.) (2007) *Competence in Social Work Practice* (2nd edn). London: Jessica Kingsley.

Orme, J. (2001) *Gender and Community Care: Social Work and Social Care Perspectives.* Basingstoke: Palgrave.

Peter, E. (2002) The history of nursing in the home: revealing the significance of place in the expression of moral agency. *Nursing Inquiry*, 9(2): 65–72.

Phillips, J., Ray, M. and Marshall, M. (2006) *Social Work with Older People* (4th edn). Basingstoke: Palgrave Macmillan.

Putnam, R. (2000) *Bowling Alone: The Collapse and Revival of American Community.* New York: Simon Shuster.

Quinney, A. (2006) *Collaborative Practice in Social Work.* Exeter: Learning Matters.

Robson, T. (2000) *The State and Community Action.* London: Pluto Press.

SCIE (2010) *A Rough Guide to Personalisation.* Adult Services Report 20. London: Social Care Institute for Excellence.

Sines, D., Saunders, M. and Forbes-Burford, J. (2009) *Community Health Care Nursing.* Chichester: Wiley-Blackwell.

Stuart-Hamilton, I. (2006) *The Psychology of Ageing* (4th edn). London: Jessica Kingsley.

Taylor, B. (2010) *Professional Decision-Making in Social Work Practice.* Exeter: Learning Matters.

Thompson, N. (2007) *Power and Empowerment.* Lyme Regis: Russell House.

Thompson, S. (2007) *Age Discrimination.* Lyme Regis: Russell House.

Titterton, M. (2005) *Risk and Risk Taking in Health and Social Welfare.* London: Jessica Kingsley.

Waine, B., Tunstill, J., Meadows, P. and Peel, M. (2005) *Developing Social Care: Values and Principles.* London: Social Care Institute for Excellence.

White, K. (2009) *An Introduction to the Sociology of Health and Illness* (2nd edn). London: Sage Publications.

Responsibilities and Accountabilities in Interprofessional Working

Hazel Colyer

Introduction

While earlier chapters have looked at challenges of managing risk with specific client groups in the current social and political context, this chapter assesses the impact of this on the development of multiple professions and interprofessional working. This is a loose term that is taken to cover the planning of interventions or care in multidisciplinary team meetings (MDT) and its delivery, either successively by different professions or concurrently in interprofessional teams. This way of working has led to improvements in outcomes for many patients and clients but it also poses challenges to the identity and autonomy of professional practitioners in terms of responsibilities and accountabilities (Milburn and Walker 2009).

Working interprofessionally is challenging for professionals but essential for quality care. Understanding the sources and scope of these challenges is helpful and, since many of them are structural, the chapter advocates the need for professionals to develop strategies that promote the safer integration of different perspectives, manage risk and mitigate any negative effects on their own professional authority.

Using cancer care as an example, I show how governance frameworks in health and social care services can weigh heavily on practitioners, making it more difficult to trust others to co-deliver care and interventions for which they are jointly accountable. At the same time, the wishes of patients and clients must be prioritised in the decision-making process and this challenges professionals to support risk-taking through enabling others.

LEARNING OUTCOMES

By the end of the chapter you should have developed your understanding of:

■ Ways of interprofessional working and challenges to professional autonomy

■ Sources of professional decision making; models, values, cultures

■ Differential responsibilities and accountabilities to self, others, patients and clients

■ Communication barriers, the significance of structural and organisational systems

■ Strategies for managing differences.

Ways of interprofessional working and challenges to professional autonomy

The need to work with others to deliver the best care is integral to modern health and social care practice for reasons that should be obvious but have needed to be constantly restated in government White Papers over the past 20 years; most recently in *Equity and Excellence, Liberating the Talents* (Department of Health 2010). This document privileges patient choice and improving outcomes above all, inferring a lesser role for specific professional interests.

In caring for people with cancer, the range of interventions available has increased greatly over the past 50 years and, in many instances, cancer is no longer the incurable death sentence that it once was. It is rare that no intervention is possible and pathways of care have been developed for every cancer site. Acute cancer care or oncology embraces surgery, radiotherapy and chemotherapy and many patients are offered all of these in the primary phase of clinical management of their disease. The key professional groups involved are oncologists (surgical, medical and radiation/clinical), therapeutic radiographers, medical physicists and specialist nurses. Every patient diagnosed with cancer should have their case discussed at the MDT, a multidisciplinary team meeting where the treatment plan is determined.

The emergence of the MDT is relatively recent and its purpose is to ensure that cancer patients are offered the best possible treatment option rather than being offered the intervention favoured by the consultant medical practitioner that they first meet. However, recent evidence suggests this may be problematic from several perspectives (Taylor *et al.* 2010). Additionally, most MDTs are doctor-led and often dominated by surgeons, they do not always include other professionals and they rarely, if ever, include patients (Fosker and Dodwell 2010).

That cancer is now regarded as a long-term condition (LTC) is evident from the publication of the NHS Cancer Plan (Department of Health 2004a). This advocates a tiered approach to care beginning with support for self-management, through to complex, multi-professional case management approaches. The development of the hospice movement and palliative medicine and care means that good quality, multiprofessional services, involving a wide range of different professionals from physiotherapists to chaplains, are available for the terminally ill and dying (Department of Health 2008).

CHALLENGE

Think about your own experience of how treatment plans or interventions are decided, either in an MDT or case conference.

■ Are the relevant professionals present?

■ Is the patient or client usually present?

■ Whose voice is the most dominant and influential?

■ What might be the obstacles to the patient or client being offered the correct treatment or intervention?

When considering these questions you may like to reflect upon earlier chapters and the rights of the patient and service user in these situations, and the responsibilities of the professionals involved towards the person concerned.

The number of regulated professions has increased dramatically since 1960 when the Council for Professions Supplementary to Medicine was set up to regulate radiography and the therapy professions. Before that time, regulation through registration applied only to nursing, midwifery, medicine, dentistry and a small number of others. In 2011, the number of occupational groups queuing to apply to join the family of 12 professions regulated by the Health Professions Council (HPC) continues to grow. The role of the HPC is to protect the public, and to regulate the education and training of professionals, it maintains a public register of properly qualified members of all the professions concerned.

There is seemingly a direct relationship between the range of health interventions and examinations and the number of professions that have emerged to undertake them. The process of professionalisation has been observed and documented by Larson (1977) and others in the following way; specialisation of work tends to lead to the emergence of an occupational group, the adoption of specific curriculum for training and a code of conduct. This may be followed by the formation of a professional association to pursue recognition and thence to an application for registration, which is the ultimate goal, since it reserves the work of the group to those who can use the registered title. An excellent example of this is the emergence during the 1950s of therapeutic radiography as a specific group within radiography, whose specialism is the management and treatment of cancer using ionising radiations. Public legitimisation of this process of professionalisation occurred in a UK parliamentary statement in the early 1990s (Lord Benson 1992) and, *inter alia,* this has led to the emergence of Operating Department Practitioners and Paramedics as examples of professional groups that have achieved registered status with the HPC since 2000.

A different model of professionalisation can be seen in the regulation of social work from 2005. This model emphasises protection of the public and, arguably, is the reason why health and social care professions have been permitted to proliferate. Prior to the setting up of the General Social Care Council (GSCC), social work was unregulated and many of the workforce were unqualified or had different standards of professional qualification. Protection of the social work title through registration has improved the status of the profession but, more importantly from the government's perspective, it has defined the threshold standards of knowledge, skills and behaviours expected of social workers in pursuance of improvements to social services. However, the Government's Health and Social Care Act (Department of Health 2011) stipulates the abolition of the GSCC and a change of name for the HPC to Health and Care Professionals Council (HCPC), requiring social workers to be registered with the HCPC in order to practise in England as a social worker.

A consequence of successful professionalisation is the claim to autonomy made by those who are members of regulated professions; this and related concepts are explored further below. The point being made here is that the rise of multiple professions, each of which lays claim to a particular area of expertise, entails commitment to interprofessional working that is a feature of modern health and social care practice.

The need for collaboration between health and social care practitioners is partly a function of the rise in the number of professions and partly a result of the increasing complexity of health and social care practices. Potentially it creates fault lines in the care pathway and, significantly, it is also a source of much criticism by patients and clients, who often experience the lack of interprofessional work as poor quality care. The fault lines that have appeared between professions occasionally make the headlines, such as the case of Baby Peter Connelly. More often, they cause unacceptable delays in treatment plans resulting in frustration and anger. In the case of newly diagnosed cancer, such delays could make the difference between being cured or not (O'Rourke and Edwards 2000).

There are two main ways of viewing how professionals can work together to deliver optimal care, linear and concurrent. The present vogue is for the construction of care as a pathway and to describe patients and clients as being 'on a journey'. During this linear journey patients may have contact with many different professionals and there are specific handover points from one type of service to another. Such referrals, as they are known, have been and in some instances, remain a potential source of conflict, since the right to refer to another professional is integral to professional status and autonomy. Historically, doctors have reserved this right to themselves and thus structural delays are built into the system through the time-consuming processes of making referrals and/or delegating the authority for care and interventions to others.

Within the patient care pathway there are also many episodes of care that demand concurrent, collaborative working among professionals. For example, preparing for a course of radiotherapy treatment entails close interprofessional working among radiographers, medical physicists and doctors, with a high level of trust between them. Any lack of trust will result in team members not 'risk-ing' the necessary sharing of responsibility that ensures that patients receive seamless and efficient care. For example, a radiotherapy treatment plan, which is a complex arrangement of radiation fields designed to produce a targeted dose distribution, may be produced by a specialist radiographer and signed off by a physicist. If the latter insisted on double checking the whole process then a delay in starting treatment could easily result.

Collaborative working may fail if members of the interprofessional team do not acknowledge the others' autonomy, expressed in respect and trust. It is useful to consider the basis on which respect for the autonomy of the other is a legitimate demand. In Chapter 1, Peter Ellis describes Hohfeld's (1919, cited in Waldron 1992) classic definitions of rights including a positive claim right that others will help you achieve something – in this case, affirmation of the other's professional autonomy and entitlement to respect.

However, there are many reasons why it may not be experienced in practice, some of which are structural and relate to hierarchy and status. In this situation, team working may be experienced as 'top down' or transactional by some members if others, often medical, believe that they should direct the activities of the team because of their historic, superior position in the social and profes-sional hierarchy. Professional hierarchies may result in some team members being unwilling to challenge others if they believe that they have greater knowl-edge than them (see Greaves and Yardley, Chapter 8). Other reasons for poor collaboration fall into the relational category, whereby an interprofessional team may fail to work collaboratively because the personalities involved are unable to promote and maintain good relationships (see also Greaves and Yardley, Chapter 8 for a discussion on 'group think' and how this can also make a signif-icant impact on decision making).

Making the transition to more effective interprofessional working in health and social care is not easy or simple as research into staff attitudes to interpro-fessional learning demonstrates (Colyer 2008). Despite espoused commitment and exposure to other professions, there is a reluctance to share responsibility with them. Building trust takes time and requires individuals to undergo (for some) an uncomfortable psycho-social transition in moving from a narrow, hierarchical, medically – dominated structure to a broader, more open, flatter team structure where trust is the essential attribute.

━━━━━━━━━━━━━━━━━━━ **CHALLENGE** ━━━━━━━━━━━━━━━━━━━

Can you name the range of professionals who might also be involved in working with your patients and clients? Identify where the major fault lines in interprofessional collaborative working may occur, and then discuss with others why these arise and how they could be avoided.

━━━

Sources of professional decision making: models, values, cultures

Decision making is a key attribute of professional autonomy and the teaching of decision-making theories and models of practice is integral to professional education programmes. For example, treatment for cancer is potentially hazardous since radiotherapy and chemotherapy doses are often at the limits of patients' physical and emotional tolerance. Mistakes have potentially catastrophic consequences for both patients and professionals. Such high-risk interventions increase the pressure on professionals, who are required to exercise high levels of professional judgement.

For interprofessional teams to be effective it is essential that the decision-making process is transparent and accepted as legitimate by the team. Thus it is pertinent to ask the questions: how do professionals make decisions about care, what sources do they use and how do they value the decisions of others?

Professional decision making is a complex process involving the interaction of knowledge, experience, values and theoretical perspectives; that is, how the professional 'views' or constructs the problem presented and the risks associated with the decisions taken. An example of this is the management of physical disability, say losing part of a leg as result of being shot in a war situation. Undoubtedly the injured person would be cared for by a number of different professionals. However, different professional practitioners construe disability in different ways; the physiotherapist might focus on improving the function of a damaged limb and prepare the person for a prosthesis using their knowledge of neuro-muscular physiology, that is, they view the problem as a biomedical one. The occupational therapist (OT) is concerned with adaption to the environment. Their concern is to find out what activities are important to the person in order that they can fit comfortably back into their social world. In other words, the OT views disability primarily as a social issue. These differing priorities could cause debate or even conflict at a team meeting to decide the best course of action for the injured person.

━━━━━━━━━━━━━━━━━━━ **CHALLENGE** ━━━━━━━━━━━━━━━━━━━

Social versus medical approaches to disability

Using the example above, imagine a conversation between a physiotherapist and an OT about their differing priorities for the injured person.

- How might this be resolved?

- What values and theoretical perspectives does your profession espouse?

- How do they compare to those of other professions that you work with?

- Is the language that you use to talk about your profession understood by others?

When thinking about the answers to the above question you may like to remember your first day as a student health or social care professional and how you have learnt how to be identified as a nurse/social worker/radiographer/therapist.

When decision making is taught in professional education programmes, novice professionals are inducted into the values and theoretical perspectives of their discipline and learn to apply their knowledge and skills within and through this professional 'lens', building up expertise through experience. Taken together these can be said to constitute the professional culture of the specific group, where culture is defined as, 'the ideas, customs, skills and arts of a people or group that are transferred, communicated or passed along ... to a succeeding generation' (*Webster's New World College Dictionary* 2010).

The choice of decision-making models and the relative weight given to different aspects of decision making by different professions is a function of professional autonomy and culture. Thus, I would argue that professional decision making in action is the expression of particular professional expertise and necessarily opaque in some respects to members of other professions and also patients and clients. In other words, I may not understand the rationale for your decisions nor accept their validity and a potential source of conflict is opened up. In acute cancer care situations this is less likely to occur because the professions involved – doctors, physicists and radiographers – construct the intervention from a similar, biomedical perspective, although they may place a different weight on other values, such as patient involvement. When the cancer progresses and becomes terminal, a dichotomy can open up between those professionals who advocate palliative medicine – active interventions – and those whose values and culture lead them to promote palliative care and a good death.

The traditional model of decision making described above is open to the charge of subjectivity and lack of transparency. It is also seen as belonging to a time when health and social care services were paternalistic in intent and patients believed that doctors and nurses always knew best and acted in their interests; a time that is now passing. However, professional cultures and tribal behaviours are remarkably persistent and supported by the language of professional knowledge, which mystifies patients and clients and may be opaque to other professionals.

Generally it is not considered sufficiently robust to base decisions on experience alone if the underpinning source of knowledge is custom and practice. Rational decision making, based on evidence that is accessible to all, is the current dominant model and is accepted by most professionals as an important step forward in care delivery.

Evidence comes in diverse forms and there is a variety of published hierarchies of evidence (Guyatt *et al.* 2000; NHMRC 1995; Mulrow and Oxman 1997). Generally these privilege the scientific method; at the top of the hierarchy is large, meta-analyses of randomised, controlled trials, followed by other quantitative methods, qualitative approaches and, lastly, professional opinion/clinical expertise. More recently, the concept of evidence-based medicine has underpinned the emergence of the Cochrane Collaborative for systematic reviews, the Social Care Institute for Excellence (SCIE) and the National Institute for Health and Clinical Excellence (NIHCE). These organisations collectively provide evidence for successful interventions and promote best practices.

The importance of this approach in acute cancer care cannot be understated. The many advances in treatment and overall survival are due to well-constructed clinical trials. Outcomes for cancer are usually measured in terms of 5-year survival and, in the case of breast cancer; this figure has increased over the past 30 years from 30 per cent to 60 per cent due to earlier diagnosis and evidence-based combinations of chemo- and radiotherapy. However, the inbuilt objectivity of randomised clinical trials also illuminates their limitations. They can tell us the overall numbers of people likely to benefit from a specific intervention but they cannot tell you or me if we will benefit.

This illustrates the need for multiple sources of evidence and the danger or privileging one over another. Different professions tend to value sources differently and, arguably, so do patients. In general, the closer one gets to identifying and meeting the particular needs of the individual, the more likely it is that qualitative evidence will be of use in making decisions. Thus, the widespread availability of evidence supports greater participation of patients in decision making.

Successive government policy documents have attempted to shift the balance of power between patients and professionals in favour of patients and a person-centred approach. Adams, in Chapter 3, explored the shifts in responsibility between the state and the individual; the shifting balance of power between patients and professionals has occurred in parallel with this but not entirely as a consequence of the policies. The many examples of poor interprofessional working, both anecdotal and from high-profile inquiries such as the serious case review on baby Peter Connolly and the Bristol Children's Hospital Inquiry, suggests that in reality this change is having only limited success. The accessibility of evidence, coupled with an internet-savvy generation, has led to many, but not all, patients demanding greater involvement in decisions about their care and a new role for professional practitioners, empowerment.

Empowerment is characterised by support for patient decision making through the interpretation of evidence and a non-judgemental approach to the outcome. Hickey and Kipping (1998) identified a participation continuum to describe the relationship between professional practitioners and patients. It begins with information/explanation and proceeds to consultation, partnership and, finally, user-control. Hickey and Kipping describe the former two as a consumerist approach and the latter as active citizenship through a process of democratisation. They suggest that professionals must adjust their practices to embrace an empowerment approach if they are to succeed in the aspiration to genuinely involve patients and clients in decision making.

For many types of breast cancer the evidence suggests that a combination of surgery, chemotherapy and radiotherapy provides the optimal treatment. Chemotherapy is a systemic treatment with many unpleasant side effects and potential long-term risks. Occasionally, having reviewed the risks and discussed them with professionals, patients may refuse to have the recommended chemotherapy. This 'informed decision' must be respected by all of the oncology team but it is often the case that some members are frustrated by the patient's decision and conflict arises among the team because of the differing weight given to the rights claim of the patients by professionals.

Given the process of professionalisation identified above, the differences in values and cultures, and the relative social positions of health care professions, this transition in role from paternalistic to partnership is difficult to achieve and is occurring at a different pace in different professions. The Health and Social Care Act (Department of Health 2011) will shift service commissioning responsibilities to groups of general practitioners (GPs) and one reason given for this is their intimate knowledge of their patients' needs. It is believed that this will 'lift' patient involvement with decision making to a societal level and make the phrase 'No decision about me without me' a greater reality.

Differential responsibilities and accountabilities to self and others

Utilitarian philosophy is based on a form of psychological egoism that asserts that the individual's own interests are necessarily more important than the interests of others (Bentham 1789). In other words, we are designed to put our own interests first and acting in the interests of the other is also ultimately self-serving. Acting out of self-interest in a professional (and ethical) context is expressed appropriately in the taking of professional responsibility for our work. As individual professional practitioners we are accountable to ourselves and others for the quality of the care and interventions that we offer. When that falls below the standards expected, then we are rightly judged by our peers and may be found guilty of misconduct or incompetence.

Accountability has been usefully framed within four pillars for nurses and midwives by Caulfield (2005, cited in Jasper 2006). These pillars, which are equally applicable to other health and social professionals, are professional, ethical, law and employment. Professional relates to published standards of professional practice by professional and statutory bodies, ethical derives from social values and individual moral codes, the civil and criminal law governs all practice, and contracts of employment set out roles, responsibilities, authorities and expectations of individual posts.

Savage and Moore's (2004) ethnographic study of how practice nurses understand accountability revealed that the term is ambiguous and that, especially in the context of the multidisciplinary team when role boundaries may become blurred, its meaning and attribution is poorly understood. In the study, which took place in one large general practice, accountability for clinical decision making was frequently referred back to the GP partners and this was exacerbated by clinical governance processes and the fear of litigation. This suggests that accountability and willingness to take and own decisions may not be as strong among some individuals and professional groups as others. There may be a tendency in multiprofessional teams for accountability for difficult decisions to be passed around like a hot potato among the members if the instinct for self-preservation comes to the fore. This raises the issue of risk appetite and how successfully education programmes that prepare practitioners for entry to one of the health and social care registers develop the ability to assess and manage risk. The selection process for doctors includes the assessment of decision-making ability and it is apparent to most health and social care practitioners that doctors do expect to take decisions. However, I have observed that some among my own profession of therapeutic radiography, whilst claiming the status of professional, are less willing to assume the responsibilities and accountability that goes with it (Colyer 2010).

Conversely, an over-strong commitment to accountability among professionals in health and social care may be a barrier to interprofessional working if they do not accept the professional status and autonomy of others. Earlier in the chapter the process of professionalisation, its relationship to autonomy and the need to respect the autonomy of the other was described. The autonomy of specific professional groups is related to a defined scope of practice, the limits of which are potentially contestable as boundaries are blurred.

As therapeutic radiographers have developed their claim to full professional status, they have sought to define their scope of practice broadly in relation to the management and delivery of the non-medical aspects of the radiotherapy process from planning to post-treatment follow-up. In health care teams, the achievement of full professional status is not yet acknowledged by all; within the medical profession, there are many who believe that only they have full clinical responsibility and therefore authority over all aspects of patient care. This responsibility for authority over the process may be delegated to the other if the lead clinician so chooses but it is never abandoned.

When clinical oncologists, physicists and radiographers work together to plan and treat a patient with cancer, this may not be a genuine collaboration among autonomous professionals with each respecting the autonomy and trusting the authority of the other. Rather, the clinical oncologist, by not accepting the authority of the radiographer and/or physicist seeks to direct the work of the others. The effect of this can be to introduce unnecessary delays in starting treatment – readers are familiar with 'waiting for the doctor' – but it can also lead to a poorer quality service. Increasing complexity and technological developments mean that it is difficult, if not impossible, for one professional to have expertise across all aspects of the radiotherapy treatment process and this is no less true in other care settings.

It is useful to consider the concept of user responsibility at this point since there is often a paradox between rights claims made by individuals in respect of their health care needs and willingness to accept responsibility, what Selbourne (1994) has termed 'dutiless rights'. It is also the case that many patients and clients are reluctant to participate in decisions about their care and treatment. In relation to public health, successive governments have sought to move from a socio-material explanatory context for poor health and health inequalities to an individual-psychological explanation. In other words, the state is not responsible for your health, you are! (see Adams in Chapter 3) and the choices you make are the main determinants. This is a highly contested area for debate as earlier chapters in this book illustrate (for example see Ellis, Chapter 1 and Bungay, Chapter 2). However, we can draw some common understandings; namely, that a right, however derived, entails a responsibility or duty, either from others or from oneself. If I believe that I have a claim right to good health and health care then I have a duty to promote it by cooperating with those who provide services.

Supporting patients and clients to participate fully in decisions about their care is difficult to achieve. In Chapter 2, Bungay explores the issues of communication and the difference in levels of knowledge between the general public and professionals. There is also a substantial imbalance of power between professional practitioners and those who use services, which must be acknowledged before it can be interrogated. It tends to create deference and an unwillingness to question the judgement of the professional. In a multiprofessional case conference, that imbalance may be even more pronounced as the patient or client is numerically overwhelmed.

================================ **CHALLENGE** ================================

■ Why do you think that some patients and clients are reluctant to become fully involved in making decisions about their care or treatment?

■ What strategies might be used to engage involvement in the decision making process?

You may like to consider the influence of age, gender, culture, and social class and levels of educational attainment when exploring how potential barriers to involvement may be overcome.

Communication barriers, the significance of structural and organisational systems

I have outlined above how the rise of multiple professions entails effective collaborative working through putting patients' needs first. However, it is also the case that different ways of professional decision making may introduce inherent communication difficulties among different professions. Research evidence about effective team working suggests that shared goals, effective communication and respect for the autonomy of the other are major determinants of good team working (Poulton and West 1999).

Good communication is about the capacity to moderate and adjust language in order to create understanding among professionals and ensure that communication with patients and clients is optimal (Sumison and Lenucha 2009). Whilst it is acknowledged that each profession has a specialist language and individual philosophies of teamwork, which enables shorthand communication to occur quickly and easily, the effect of this on other team members may be to exclude them from conversations. This mystification could sometimes be perceived as deliberate exclusion in order to maintain boundaries and keep professional hierarchies in place.

Poor or absent communication is at the heart of most failures to provide the appropriate care or intervention across the patient pathway. The fault lines between professionals referred to above are often exacerbated by organisational structures that are not aligned, information systems that do not 'speak' to each other and an insistence by some practitioners on keeping individual records rather than shared record keeping. These structural fault lines are especially apparent between statutory health and social care services due to their different governance arrangements and funding streams. Added complications can occur when the voluntary sector is involved.

An example of this is services for people with terminal cancer, where 50 per cent of care is provided by the charitable hospice sector and the challenge of working interprofessionally is great. A terminally ill person may be under the care of the cancer centre, primary health care practitioners, the hospice and local social services at the same time. One way of alleviating some of the communication barriers inherent in this scenario and modelling patient-centredness is the case management model, where one professional takes the lead in supporting the patient to navigate the complexities (Department of Health 2004b). This solution also mitigates the risks inherent in such a complex situation.

Developing strategies to overcome differences and maximise interprofessional working

This chapter has attempted to analyse and explain some of the challenges faced by professionals in health and social care in doing their jobs in a multiprofessional environment. These challenges go to the heart of what it means to be a modern professional in a complex environment where boundaries are not always clearly defined and risk management is an ever-present reality of daily practice.

The challenges concern the imperative to be person-centred, the increasing number of occupational groups involved, the range of settings in which care and treatments is offered and the technological complexity of available interventions. They demand professionals who are able to differentiate responsibilities, manage risk and be accountable in uncertain situations.

While this requires a high level of knowledge and skills, managing the process of working collaboratively also demands a high level of social competence, interpersonal skills and empathy. Emotional intelligence (EI) is a term coined by Savoley and Mayer (1990: 189) who define it as 'a form of social intelligence that involves the ability to monitor one's own and others emotions, to discriminate among them and use this information to guide one's thinking and actions'. It is suggested that EI is a personality trait and that therefore the level differs in individuals (Goleman 1995).

It may be that individuals have differing amounts of emotional intelligence at the point of entry to professional education programmes. However, a vital aspect of professional development concerns insight and reflection leading to professional maturity. Focusing on this in professional preparation programmes and continuing professional development is an important means of enhancing collaborative competence. When we understand the impact of our behaviour and actions on others and theirs on us, we can better manage the dynamics in teams.

In conclusion, some of the structural barriers to working interprofessionally will not easily be solved and so must be factored into our thinking when planning services. This raises the importance of acknowledging the inherent risks in interprofessional working in order that they can be faced and policies developed that mitigate them. For professionals to be effective collaborative practitioners in empowering partnerships with patients and clients there is a need for a new transparency and honesty about the scale of the challenge, a desire to cultivate the professional maturity to be accountable and a willingness to share the risks.

CHALLENGE

Thinking about your own practice and the responsibilities and accountabilities in interprofessional working, consider the following:

■ How do I balance professional accountability with the need to work collaboratively with others?

■ What is the relative contribution of personal and professional attributes to working effectively with others?

■ What strategies might be useful in overcoming structural obstacles to respectful working with others?

It is helpful to have a brief example of good practice to help think about the benefits and potential difficulties in relation to multiprofessional working from the perspective of service users and carers. Working with a gentleman, Mr A who had been diagnosed at the age of 60 with motor neurone disease, a very serious neurological condition that paralyses the body – often leading to swallowing and choking difficulties, incontinence, mobility and communication difficulties –but which leaves the mind unaffected, there was a well-established multidisciplinary team from the local hospice including the consultant, the nurse, the occupational therapist, the speech therapist and the social worker. They all knew each other's roles and communication was good. They had worked together on a number of very difficult cases and most of them were physically based at the hospice where interprofessional working is often seen at its best (Leathard 2003).

There was a multidisciplinary discussion where the professionals discussed the situation and made plans for their interventions. They knew that it often took about two years from diagnosis to the terminal stages of the disease but there were cases where people could remain relatively well for a number of years. Hoping the progress of the disease would be not too rapid in this case, the group decided at the first meeting not to unduly alarm Mr and Mrs A by giving them too much information about the prognosis, although they were given verbal information about some of the services available to them. The team then wrote to Mr A inviting him to contact them again when he felt he needed further assistance. Rather than imposing their views and services, the team felt that in this way they were handing the responsibility over to Mr A and his family for when they felt they were ready to access services.

Both Mr A and his wife had to give up work so she could look after him and there were some financial difficulties. Mrs A contacted the local social services and a community care manager called to discuss these issues and found the couple very distressed. Mrs A said she knew all these people were involved but she didn't know who she should contact about what; she couldn't remember people's names and as a result she felt she was unable to do her best to help her husband. The community care manager had to admit that she didn't really know who did what in this interprofessional team either, so she organised a multidisciplinary meeting in the service user's home. Each of the professionals introduced themselves to Mr and Mrs A, wore a name badge and gave a short speech about her role. At the end of the meeting, Mrs A and the care manager got together and drew up a chart with the names of all the professionals, alongside their contact details and a synopsis of their roles and responsibilities.

This example shows how with the best will in the world it is not always possible for practitioners to know what is best for people who use services. Interprofessional working and professional accountability are undoubtedly important topics for practitioners but genuine collaborative working will never really address the tensions between rights, risks and responsibilities unless service users, and carers, are fully involved in the process.

References

Benson, Lord (1992) *The Professions*. Official Report 5th Series. Parliamentary Debates 1992–93, Lords vol. 538, Gun 15, 9 July 1992: 1208–1210. London: Hansard.

Bentham, J. (1789) *An Introduction to the Principles of Morals and Legislation*, cited in J. S. Mill (1982) *Utilitarianism*. Glasgow: Collins.

Colyer, H. (2008) Embedding interprofessional learning in pre-registration education in health and social care: evidence of cultural lag. *Learning in Health and Social Care*, 7(3): 126–33.

Colyer, H. (2010) Therapeutic Radiography at the crossroads: guest editorial. *Radiography*, 16: 3–4. Available at: http://dx.doi.org/10.1016/j.radi.2009.10.009.

Department of Health (2004a) *The NHS Cancer Plan and the New NHS: Providing a Patient-centred Service*. London: The Stationery Office.

Department of Health (2004b) *Supporting People with Long Term Conditions*. London: The Stationery Office.

Department of Health (2008) *End of Life Care Strategy*. London: The Stationery Office.

Department of Health (2010) *Equity and Excellence: Liberating the Talents*. London: The Stationery Office.

Department of Health (2011) *The Health and Social Care Act*. London: The Stationery Office.

Fosker, C. and Dodwell, D. (2010) The cost of the MDT. Available at: http://www.bmj.com/content/340/bmj.c951.extract/reply (accessed 7 March 2011).

Goleman, D. (1995) *Emotional Intelligence: Why it Can Matter More Than IQ*. New York: Bantam Books.

Guyatt, G. H., Haynes, R. B., Jaeschke, R. Z., Cook, D. J., Green, L., Naylor, C. D., Wilson, M. C. & Richardson, W. S. (2000) Users' guide to the medical literature XXV. Evidence-based medicine: Principles for applying the users guides to patient care. *JAMA*, 284(10): 1290–96.

Hickey, G. and Kipping, C. (1998) Exploring the concept of user involvement in mental health through a participation continuum. *Journal of Clinical Nursing*, 7(1): 83–8.

Jasper, M. (2006) *Vital Notes for Nurses: Professional Development, Reflection and Decision Making*. Oxford: Blackwell.

Larson, M. S. (1977) *The Rise of Professionalism: A Sociological Analysis*. Berkeley, CA: University of California Press.

Leathard, A. (ed.) (2003) *Interprofessional Collaboration: From Policy to Practice in Health and Social Care*. Hove: Brunner-Routledge.

Milburn, P. and Walker, P. (2009) Beyond interprofessional education and towards collaborative person-centred practice. In G. Koubel and H. Bungay (eds), *The Challenge of Person-centred Care: An Interprofessional Perspective*. Basingstoke: Palgrave Macmillan.

Mulrow, C. D. and Oxman, A. D. (1997) *Cochrane Collaboration Handbook* (database on disk and CD-ROM). The Cochrane Library, The Cochrane Collaboration, Oxford, Updated Software.

NHMRC (1995) *Guidelines for the Development and Implementation of Clinical Guidelines*, 1st edn. Canberra: Australian Government Publishing Service.

O'Rourke, N. and Edwards, R. (2000) Lung cancer treatment waiting times and tumour growth. *Clinical Oncology*, 12: 141–4.

Poulton, B. and West, M. (1999) The determinants of effectiveness in primary health care teams. *Journal of Interprofessional Care*, 13: 7–18.

Savage, J. and Moore, L. (2004) *Interpreting Accountability: An Ethnographic Study of Practice Nurses Accountability and Multidisciplinary Team Decision Making in the Context of Clinical Governance*, Royal College of Nursing Institute Research Report. Available at: www.rcn.org.uk (accessed 14 February 2011).

Savoley, P. and Mayer, J. D. (1990) Emotional intelligence. *Imagination, Cognition and Personality*, 9: 185–211.

Selbourne, D. (1994) *The Principle of Duty*. London: Sinclair-Stevenson.

Sumison, T. and Lenucha, R. (2009) Therapists' perceptions of how teamwork influences client-centred practice. *British Journal of Occupational Therapy*, 72(2): 48–54.

Taylor, C., Munro, A., Glynne-Jones, R., Griffith, C., Trevatt, P., Richards, M. and Ramirez, A. (2010) Multidisciplinary team working in cancer: what is the evidence? *British Medical Journal*, 340. Available at: http://www.bmj.com/content/340/bmj.c951 (accessed 7 March 11).

Waldron, J. (1992) 'Introduction'. In J. Waldron (ed.), *Theories of Rights*. Oxford: Oxford University Press.

Webster's New World College Dictionary (2010) Cleveland, OH: Wiley (accessed online 18 February 2011).

Critical Reflections on Balancing Rights, Risks and Responsibilities

Georgina Koubel

Introduction

The chapter explores different models for understanding disability, risk and vulnerability. Recognising the importance of a measured and integrated model for managing the complex balance in cases involving rights, risks and responsibilities, I propose a reflective or process model of practice which can enable practitioners to be prepared to deal with complexity and uncertainty that inform these challenging dilemmas. Models of disability, vulnerability, partnership and power will help us to understand and manage the process of risk in the interprofessional arena.

There are opportunities for exploration and analysis of the relationship between professional responsibilities and person-centred care in complex situations of risk involving vulnerable people, as well as reflections on the different values different professionals and practitioners may bring to the process of decision making in relation to adults perceived as vulnerable and at risk. Examining interprofessional perspectives and discourses, the chapter will look at the application of a reflective, process model of risk and analyse its value for working in situations of complexity and uncertainty. There are reflective exercises in the form of challenges, and analysis of a complex case study scenario to enable readers to engage in critical reflection on personal and professional attitudes to risk and consider the implications of these for practice in health and social care.

An integrated model of practice is presented, which I have called the PREPARED model; it is based on social perspectives and values around anti-discriminatory practice (Thompson 2007) but as it is person-centred it will be equally relevant for practitioners across the realm of health as in social care. The purpose of this model is to provide a framework for working in complex situations involving the balance of rights, risks and responsibilities.

LEARNING OUTCOMES

By the end of the chapter you should have developed your understanding of:

■ Your own attitudes to risk, and to your own and others' safety

■ Discourses on disability, power, professional responsibility and danger and their relevance to the assessment of risk

■ Social models of empowerment and vulnerability and their challenge to procedural notions of safeguarding, vulnerability and risk for people with disabilities

■ The balance of rights, risks and responsibilities in relation to personal autonomy, mental capacity and professional decision making

■ The integration of a reflective or process model for practice that can be applied when working in complex situations involving vulnerable people, their carers and the wider community.

Within the context of health and social care there is a place for technical models of risk analysis and decision making that can take account of the critical nature of the work but there is a difference in the ways in which models of risk assessment can be applied to, for example, clinical treatments or social work interventions. Practitioners from diverse disciplines need to be aware of these so that they can contribute their perspectives in order to make secure and accountable decisions.

However, there are many other situations within health and social care where the power of professionals to influence or even overpower the views and wishes of service users may become abusive in itself. While understanding the need for decisive and even urgent action in some situations, a process or reflective model of risk highlights the variety of elements that contribute to professional judgments and decisions in practice (Jasper 2006). Using a reflective model of practice that encompasses issues of risk but which also considers the rights, roles and responsibilities of the various stakeholders involved can help to develop a considered, systematic, critical and person-centred approach to the understanding, assessment and management of complex risky situations.

CHALLENGE

What models of risk assessment are you familiar with, either from your reading or your practice? Identify one to analyse further: if you haven't used one before, you could choose one of the models highlighted in Chapter 4.

■ What do you think are the principles that underpin the model you have selected?

■ What do you think are the good things about this model?

■ What do you think are the limitations of the model?

All models, however well developed, will have advantages and drawbacks. One argument may be that practitioners may not always have the time to carry out a systematic risk assessment, and the important thing is to ensure the person is safe. This may at times contravene some people's human rights, and as we have identified this is particularly likely in situations where people are perceived as vulnerable. There are certainly a range of situations where safeguarding procedures are required to protect vulnerable children and adults from harm, and when these are not carried out effectively the consequences can be tragic. The findings from a number of serious case reviews have identified the failings of various professionals to take the appropriate action and places emphasis on the responsibilities of practitioners from health and social care to improve their practice in these areas. What may be less clear in these cases is how practitioners weighed the balance between rights and risks, and how they understood their responsibilities towards people who are deemed to be vulnerable.

Discourses on disability and vulnerability

It is important to acknowledge that many of the concepts we have discussed throughout this book are contingent, that is they change and their significance varies depending on the ideological and political perspectives of those who make and influence policy. These 'constantly shifting power relationships between state, service users and health care and social work professionals' (Johns 2007) raise particular challenges around professional judgements and decision making in relation to people at risk.

In analysing and planning to manage situations of risk, the assessment skills and ethical frameworks of the person carrying out the assessment will be of particular importance. Swain *et al.* (2005) make the point that although the medical model of disability which labels disabled people as unfit, sick or incapable may be becoming less prevalent, the tragedy model which paints the picture of disabled people as brave victims who desperately need help from the able-bodied society is one that is instantly recognisable from charity appeals. The social model, which recognises the strengths and rights of the person with disabilities, turns these models around and labels society as the disabling factor because it fails to make the necessary accommodations to enable people with disabilities to participate fully in the social mainstream. There are further writers such as Morris (1997) who suggest there is a need for a more subtle integration of the issues of impairment and disability purely as social construct.

The value of understanding these different views in the context of rights, risks and responsibilities is that they affect the way we interpret and understand the world, and these then affect the way we picture in our mind people who are described as vulnerable. If a medical or tragedy model is our main model of understanding disability (or age), this will affect the way services are provided and the manner in which professionals react to service users, seeing them only in terms of people who are unfortunate and needing help. The risk is that this may lead to attitudes that are patronising or dismissive of people's ability to make their own choices and decisions.

Although the Mental Capacity Act 2005 specifically states that a person cannot be deemed incapacitated because of their age, because they have a particular medical condition or because they wish to make a decision that others may consider unwise, as we have seen in earlier chapters there is a risk to someone's autonomy, particularly if they are seen as vulnerable, because of the nature of power within relationships between those who use services and the professionals who provide them. When people are unwell or feeling overwhelmed by circumstances, which is mostly when practitioners from health and social care will encounter them, decisions may be based on the possibility of risk or harm at the expense, at times, of considering the strengths and wishes of the individual, and for a number of reasons service users may give into the wishes of others (Brown 2010).

Practitioners holding a social model of vulnerability, on the other hand, will aim to build a partnership with service users, recognising their rights and valuing and utilising their experience of their own condition as a major contribution to any decisions that are required (Martin 2007). In this context, decisions around capacity should be carefully considered, paying as much attention as possible to the value given to the views and choices of people even where they are considered vulnerable or at risk in some way. If someone is deemed not to have capacity (and, remember, this should be decision-specific and carried out only once all possible methods of enabling the person at the heart of the process to contribute as fully as possible) then there are a number of strategies for managing their affairs, including the appointment of an independent advocate if necessary.

This question of how to manage situations where adults have capacity but where they may be at risk for other reasons is one that continues to raise issues of uncertainty and anxiety. These are cases that leave practitioners in a difficult situation, concerned about the risks being run by an individual who may be being abused or exploited, or who may be neglecting themselves, but where they have no legitimate authority to intervene. Families, friends, neighbours and communities may also be very concerned and expect the social worker or care manager to intervene because of the level of risk without really taking into account the rights, wishes and choices of the individual involved. Often practitioners are left in the position of having to explain the limits of their powers and the rights of individuals to take responsibility for their own decisions if they have the capacity to do so. However, finding the right balance is not easy. Avoiding 'difficult situations' by simply assuming autonomy for vulnerable individuals may also be one way of avoiding the conflicts and dilemmas which arise from complex cases involving an uncomfortable tension between risks, rights and responsibilities, so practitioners will also need at times to engage with the exercise of authority and control when the risks appear too great.

> Indiscriminate application of the mantra of independence, choice and control in the context of self-directed care – this leaves some vulnerable adults at sometimes serious risk. (Galpin and Bates 2009: 42)

These tensions were very much apparent in the case of Steven Hoskin, whose death led to a Serious Case Review in 2007, which resulted in the local authority being severely castigated for not responding to the needs of the individual concerned. In Steven Hoskin's case, it was recognised that he met the eligibility criteria for services owing to his learning disability but once he decided not to have services anymore, the case was closed without any further risk assessment or risk management plan in place. Despite the fact that a number of people raised concerns about the people who were hanging around Steven's house, and that Steven himself went to the police on a number of occasions, there was no move to intervene to protect someone who, although he chose not to accept services, was particularly vulnerable in his need for friends and companions. Eventually, Steven was pushed off a railway bridge after months of torture and abuse at the hands of his so-called 'friends'.

In this case it was considered unacceptable for services or practitioners to simply 'wash their hands' if, for example, a vulnerable adult refuses services. In the Executive Summary by the Cornwall Adult Protection Committee of the Serious Case Review following the death of Steven Hoskin, Flynn delivered an important synopsis of the roles and responsibilities of local authorities in the context of the rights of vulnerable people, which is worth quoting at some length.

> All agencies have legal responsibilities not only to prevent harm being caused by their own agents, but to safeguard vulnerable people against the harmful actions of third parties. ... Failure to take reasonable and appropriate steps to safeguard individuals from abuse or life-threatening events is in breach of Articles 2 and 3 of the European Convention on Human Rights. It is important that adult protection is triggered when someone is *believed* to be at risk of harm/abuse and not only at the point where there is demonstrable evidence of harm. ... In order to conform to their obligations under human rights law, agencies have to be proactive in undertaking risk assessments to ensure preventative action is taken wherever practical. (Flynn 2007: 21)

Striking a balance between autonomy and vulnerability

The key dilemma in situations like this, and one which has been explored at some length in various parts of this book, is the rights of (all) adults to determine their own lives without undue interference from the state, even at risk of exploitation and abuse. England has decided (partly through the *No Secrets*

Consultation Process, Department of Health 2009) not to bring in any further legal remedies for adults at risk but in Scotland there is a different law which does allow intervention in cases where people with capacity are at risk but unable to take action because they are believed to be under the power or influence of someone else.

Purely rational decision making would mean that none of us would stay in relationships that are harmful to us, or let people exploit or abuse us. However, if we take time to think about it, we know that we do not always act in this reasonable, calm, calculated way. We often know what we (or someone else) should do but do something else because of a measure of emotional dependence. The Scottish legislation, the Adult Support and Protection Act 2007, which came into force in autumn 2008, recognises that these may be the very times when legal intervention may be appropriate, if not essential. This Act gives the local authority powers to carry out an investigation, as available to practitioners in England under the *No Secrets* guidance (Department of Health 2000), but it also enables the practitioner in Scotland to apply to a court for an Assessment Order to remove the individual for an assessment of whether they are likely to experience significant harm, a Removal Order to remove the person to a specific place to protect them from being seriously harmed, or a Banning Order to prevent a particular person having contact with the adult at risk. The Act requires the person at risk to agree to these terms in most circumstances.

However – and this is the significant difference from the remedies available to practitioners in England – under the Scottish legislation, the court can decide to impose these orders if they believe that 'the adult at risk has been unduly pressurized [or] there are no steps which could reasonably be taken with the adult's consent which would protect the adult from the harm which the order or action is intended to prevent' (Armstrong 2008: 69).

Many practitioners who have worked with vulnerable adults have at times wished they had these powers which would enable them to protect adults who despite the level of risk, or even harm, that they are enduring decides not to accept help or intervention and who are deemed to have the capacity to make this decision. However, it does raise questions about the limit to the ultimate choices and wishes of any one of us as citizens and autonomous individuals. Which is more important to you – the absolute rights to your own and others' self-determination and autonomy or the right of the state to take action if you (or someone else who may be deemed vulnerable but who has mental capacity) decide to take unjustifiable risks? Or is it more complicated than that? Have a look at the Challenge that follows and carefully consider your reactions, values and responses. Then think about how these relate to notions of rights, risks and responsibilities in working with vulnerable people.

CHALLENGE

You see a couple arguing in the street across the road from where you are walking. They are both shouting but then the man hits the woman quite hard and she starts crying. It is possible they have both been drinking. What (if anything) would you do?

This is a situation which could set any of us calculating the balance of probabilities on quite an instinctive level. Issues of risk, to yourself as well as the other parties involved, will be passing through your brain: if I say something, what are the chances he could end up hitting me? If that's the case, how big and strong does he look? Could I get seriously hurt? If these are the risks, what are the possible benefits of getting involved? Could I end up making things worse for the woman involved?

There are significant considerations in terms of rights and responsibilities too: do I have any right to intervene uninvited into someone else's situation? Would she welcome my intervention or see me as an interfering busybody? Is it my responsibility anyway? Are there other people around who could intervene? If so, why is it my concern rather than someone else's, or indeed everyone else's? Would other people support me if I did take action by confronting the individual involved? If not or if there's no one else around, back to the above – what are the risks to me if I do tackle the situation on my own?

Other factors that will affect your response will be your own values, attitudes and previous experiences. Here are a few further questions to ask yourself:

■ Would I react differently if this incident involved people I already knew?

■ Would I react differently if the 'victim' was obviously vulnerable (for example if she were a child, an older woman or someone with a visible disability)? What would I do in that situation?

■ Would I react differently in my role as a professional if this attack occurred in my place of work?

So the way we calculate actions, even in a situation where we do not have much time to consciously apply any risk assessment models, involves both rational and emotional responses and an ability to weigh up the consequences of different modes of action very quickly. This of course does not mean that we always feel we made the right decision. At times we may feel afterwards that we overreacted, or that our intervention was ill-judged, ineffective or unwelcome. If we did nothing we may feel guilty that we did not react in the way we would like to think our principles would guide us. We may make judgements about the consequences of our action or non-intervention in private life; the difference of course in professional judgement is that we can be held accountable for our behaviour by others (Jasper 2006), and therefore need to be able to 'give account' of the reasons for the way in which we reacted.

In a professional setting it is not really acceptable to do nothing, unless we can demonstrate the reasons for non-intervention. Regarding the incident outlined above, we may quite reasonably deem that it would be too dangerous on a personal level to physically intervene but in professional practice we would need to demonstrate how and why we had made that decision, and also show that we had done whatever we could to help the individual. However, this does not give us the right to make decisions on her behalf. We may be able to provide evidence (by carefully recording conversations, for example), that we persuaded someone experiencing domestic violence to get medical attention and seek legal advice and even to leave the person who attacked her to go and stay in a refuge. Recording is an important requirement for practitioners. At a later stage for any number of reasons (some we may not even be aware of) she may decide she does not want to take action against the party who assaulted her, or she may decide to go back to live with him, fully aware of the dangers involved. If the woman were considered vulnerable because of age, ill health or because she had a disability we may be able to call on safeguarding procedures (Association of Directors of Adult Services 2005). However, this does not negate someone's rights to self-determination.

The situation above demonstrates a number of factors that need to be taken into consideration, including the uncertainties that cannot be calculated and the fluid dynamics involved. Alongside the need for the conscious balancing of rights, risks and responsibilities within professional practice, there also has to be the recognition of the impossibility of ever getting that balance completely right. Even if it were possible to make the 'right' decision, a slight change in the system that supports the calculated risk will affect that precarious balance and may require a further level of assessment and a renegotiation of the balance among these three components. Supervision, reflection and critical self-awareness are therefore required to enable practitioners to work effectively with the complexity and uncertainties involved in risk assessment and risk management (Fook and Gardner 2010).

The following case study highlights issues of rights, risks and responsibilities and considers the factors that influence professional judgement and the models that practitioners use to resolve potential conflicts that emerge within complex practice.

CASE STUDY

When their father died two years ago, Ravi and Chandrika Vishnamurthi took on the care of Ravi's mother, Sari, who was 76 at the time, and moved her into their spacious and well-kept family home. She had recently been diagnosed with dementia and although at that time it was causing minimal disruption, her poor memory was leaving her in some risky situations such as forgetting to turn off the gas and losing keys. When a social worker had visited to offer assistance at the time, Ravi and Chandrika assured him that they considered it their responsibility to look after their mother and they did not want or need any help with this. The social worker noted that Sari looked well fed and well cared for, although he did not actually speak with her on her own, partly because of the language barrier. He used his cultural awareness and social work values to respect the wishes of the family to take on the role of carers, and did not pursue the matter further. After helping the family to fill out forms for benefits to which Sari was entitled, the social worker invited them to get in touch again if they needed any assistance in the future.

→

→

Sari was recently admitted to hospital with a urinary tract infection and the ward sister has picked up on a number of concerns which she has relayed to the care manager in the hospital. She felt that Sari was surprisingly quiet, passive and unresponsive considering the pain she must have been in. On questioning Chandrika Vishnamurthi, she discovered that that they had been giving Sari strong sleeping pills so that she did not risk harming herself by wandering around the house in the night and also keeping her more or less restricted to her room in order to manage what they found at times her 'difficult behaviour' which, Chandrika explained, put both her and Sari at risk and which additionally would not be acceptable in front of people who visited their home.

=============================== **CHALLENGE** ===============================

▨ What is your first reaction to what you have just read?

▨ Do you think perhaps the original social worker missed out on some issues that have now become apparent?

▨ If so, why do you think this happened?

▨ Are you concerned about possibilities of abuse, and if so of what kind?

The hospital care manager wonders whether the original social worker was so impressed by the material well-being of Ravi and Chandrika that he made an assumption that they would be good providers for Sari because, perhaps, they would share his personal and professional values and beliefs about Sari's best interests (Banks 2006). He may also have made the assumption that coming from an Indian family meant they would have felt that it was automatically their duty and responsibility to take care of Sari, and that they would be happy to take this on. However, it may have been that the social worker only had a very limited understanding of the Indian culture (Laird 2008), and that this superficial awareness provided a possibly erroneous level of reassurance which led him to put less priority on other values such as the rights and wishes of the individual concerned. One of the ward staff has also noticed that Sari appears to have some fingertip bruising on her arms and back. The possibility of abuse cannot be ruled out.

The ward sister has clearly spent some time thinking about the meaning of what she is seeing when she has been providing nursing care for Sari. Originally she queried the amount of medication that Sari appeared to be taking, as she is aware from attendance at a recent Adult Protection training course that overmedication could be seen as abuse. In addition her own experience of working on children's wards has led her to reflect on her practice knowledge that in working with children it was understood that a urinary tract infection could indicate possible sexual abuse, and although at this stage there is no evidence to back up this idea, she shares her concerns with the care manager who will need to take it forward in line with safeguarding or Adult Protection procedures.

Another possibility that occurs to the care manager as they discuss the issue is whether Sari is getting the money to which she is entitled, and whether this is being used for her benefit or whether the money is being subsumed into the household income which could be a form of financial abuse.

As a vulnerable adult Sari is entitled to adult protection because she is:

> An adult aged 18 years or over 'who is or may be in need of community care services by reason of mental or other disability, age or illness; and who is or may be unable to take care of him or herself, or unable to protect him or herself against significant harm or exploitation'. (Department of Health 2000)

In this case the nurse has used her knowledge and prior experience (practice wisdom) to highlight possible areas of concern. She has shared these appropriately with a colleague whose remit includes the investigation of possible adult abuse. The care manager's role is to consult with senior colleagues to decide on the best way forward. For the present Sari is in hospital and any investigation will need to be carried out in consultation with colleagues including possibly the police and health colleagues (Martin 2007). It is important that this process is carried out in a careful and systematic way. Assumptions may be wrong and evidence must be sought, and protocols dictate that, until a decision has been reached by the key professionals, no one should make the investigation of abuse more difficult by confronting the family or asking Sari any 'leading questions'. The values and principles of the practitioners involved should mean that Sari's needs, and if possible her views and wishes, should be placed firmly at the heart of any intervention (Scragg and Mantell 2011).

There are a number of possible outcomes in a situation like this. One possibility is that the fingertip bruising is being caused by the hired carers who Ravi and Chandrika have employed to help Sari with her personal care, and this may be abuse as in causing intentional harm or in that they are inadequately trained for the task. It may be that the 'difficult behaviour' that Sari is exhibiting is caused by an increase in her dementia, and that further treatment and updated guidance can help the Vishnamurthis to find alternative ways of understanding and addressing the situation. Alternatively it is possible that she is still dealing with the loss of her husband and that the 'wandering' is at least partly attributable to the fact that she was moved away from the home they had shared together within a very few weeks of his death (Currer 2007).

For many carers the pressures of looking after someone with dementia can cause friction even in close relationships and expert support and guidance from a range of professionals can help to promote the kind of person-centred care (Kitwood 1997) that could improve the family's ability to manage the difficulties involved. Any investigation has to consider the evidence, the options and in particular the wishes, choices and best interests of the adult who may be at risk.

In trying to balance the rights of Sari and her son and daughter-in-law, it is crucial that practitioners take a systematic and careful approach to the situation, trying to balance the rights, risks and responsibilities of the various stakeholders involved. The following model, which I have called the PREPARED model, provides guidance for managing complex situations when working with vulnerable people in health and social care.

PREPARED: a reflective model for integrated practice

This model is based on a notion of a number of elements which make up good, ethical practice and which makes a conscious attempt to promote the views and rights of people who come into contact with health and social care services. The model highlights the need for consciously reflective, self-aware, accountable practitioners who are trying to work sensitively and effectively in complex situations. While not underestimating the pressures practitioners encounter when working in situations of risk and uncertainty, the model should be understood within the context of the political and ideological parameters of policy which frame the relationships between the individual and the state (see Chapter 3) and which thereby affect the expectations and requirements of those undertaking professional roles and tasks within health and social work (or social care) practice. It provides a model of integrated practice that recognises complexity and uncertainty and which reflects the dilemmas and decisions faced by practitioners and integrates the experience of those using health and social care services.

'PREPARED' is an acronym of what I consider the essential features of what good professional practice should look like. Following the table, each of the headings are explored in greater detail and applied to the Case Study we have just been looking at.

P *Professional*: be aware of policies/procedures, boundaried; collaborative; careful; be critically aware of your own roles and beliefs

R *Respectful*: value differences, be aware of cultures, contexts and communication with service users, carers and colleagues

E *Evidence-based*: be up to date with knowledge, research and theoretical materials and think about how these can be applied in practice

P *Participatory*: be ethical, engage as far as possible honestly and in partnership with service users; ensure interventions are proportional and fair

A *Alert*: be active, engaged, critically aware of different accountabilities and values and their significance for positive practice

R *Reflective*: use reflection to weigh up and review rights, risks and responsibilities; use supervision or support to increase self-awareness

E *Empowering*: be aware of how professional power can support or disempower and consider the power dynamics inherent in any intervention

D *Decisive*: know when and how to be dynamic and decisive – don't just drift. This is particularly important in situations of abuse.

Professional

Professionals involved in the assessment and management of risk need to be aware of the relevant policies and procedures but not to be driven by them. They should be able to apply relevant agency directives but also to be critical of them if they do not appear to meet the needs of the service users concerned. The professional approach stresses the importance of critical practice rather than unthinkingly following (or refusing to follow) the rules. Professional practice involves constructive collaboration with colleagues, including those from other disciplines and agencies. Professional practice does not involve slavish adherence to procedures. As a professional one must be aware of the good points about one's profession – and agency – but this should not make us overly defensive about critical feedback or immune to the possibility of being wrong.

The most important element of professional practice is working *with* (not doing *to* or *for*) service users. Whether we call them patients, clients, partners, customers, citizens or service users, these are the people whose lives are affected by ill health or social problems to such an extent that they need to engage with those who provide these services. As professionals we are paid to provide those services – and we need to ensure that we do this in a way that respects the boundaries of our relationships with service users. In other words, as professionals we need to remember that those who use services are at the centre of the process, not the organisational policies and procedures that at times seem to overwhelm the essentially personal and relational nature of the work we do.

Professional practice requires a careful, measured, integrated approach even when – and perhaps especially when – emotions and work pressures could lead to hasty judgements. A professional approach requires practitioners to be fair and equitable. This is of course laudable but being human, as the case study highlighted, we also need to be critically aware of any bias or external factors that are affecting theirs' or others' practice.

Respectful

Respect is one of those words used widely in health and social care but genuinely respectful practice is not always easy to achieve (Koubel and Bungay 2009). This is partly because there is an inherent tension between the systems of health and social care and the kind of rule-bound or formulaic practice that is often used to keep those systems operational. No one who has worked in a nursing home for older people with all the demands on the staff's time, or visited someone in an acute hospital ward where no one seems to have time to talk to any of the people who are lying in bed, sick and scared, can doubt that there is an inherent pressure on staff to meet the needs of the system before the needs of the individuals who use that system. That is why the Codes of Ethics for the various governing bodies and the underpinning values of health and social care practice emphasise the importance of respect for persons (Gray and Webb 2010). The most important aspect of respect is to increase our awareness and highlight the risk of professional abuse or misuse of power as

Melville-Wiseman delineates in Chapter 7, if we lose sight of the need to respect service users. Respect is also vital for appreciating and valuing the cultural differences and different beliefs and perspectives that service users, as whole people, bring to their experience of using services (Dominelli 2002).

Relating this to the case study, the requirement for respectfulness means being aware of cultural differences but being neither dismissive of them nor bending over backwards to accommodate them. It means ensuring that Sari is treated as a person with rights and whose choices should be sought and promoted wherever possible. One key factor here is that no professional has ever tried to speak with Sari herself, and the use of an interpreter (rather than a member of the family) would give her an independent voice.

Evidence-based

Evidence-based practice in health and social care has become an increasingly significant factor informing practice and decision making in health and social care since the 1990s (Hek and Moule 2006). However, there can be differences of interpretation about what this term means in each of these settings, and it is helpful to understand what is meant by evidence-based practice and how it can inform work undertaken in relation to people who use services, and why it is considered important. Traditionally, health services have been more informed by quantitative data (random controlled trials etc.) while social work, with its more holistic approach to practice, found qualitative data more helpful. Ideally both parties should look at what data of all kinds can offer. Perhaps the most lucid explanation of the value of evidence-based practice is that it 'calls for decision making that is considered rather than reactive' (Newman *et al.* 2005: 7).

The idea of evidence may be constructed in a number of ways. In cases like the scenario discussed above, evidence may mean the physical or verbal evidence needed to support or challenge the practitioners' instinctive concerns about potential abuse, or it may be the theoretical knowledge and practice experience that each person brings to developing a hypothesis about what might be going on. In relation to the kinds of complex situations that arise in health and social care, conscientious practitioners should also seek out relevant knowledge and look at relevant research that may provide some objective guidance in the difficult process of assessment, judgement and decision making. The role of practitioners and service users (depending on key ethical considerations) being involved in practice research is also gaining ground in health and social care.

Participatory

The nature of participatory practice is the recognition of the need to be ethical, to engage honestly with service users, and to be proportional and fair in any intervention. The key principles under the Guidance that accompanies the Mental Capacity Act 2005 is that of the *assumption of capacity* unless it can be proved otherwise (which implies that practitioners should find ways to work with service users in ways which recognise their autonomy and enter into a partnership which as far as possible places the service user at the heart of the process), and the requirement that any intervention with someone who has lost capacity should be the *least restrictive possible* (Brammer 2010).

Participatory practice involves the need for any engagement and intervention with people who may be at risk or vulnerable to be firmly based on ethical principles that raise issues about autonomy, paternalism and self-determination (Bowles *et al.* 2006). Looking back at the earlier case study, it appears impossible to work in a participatory way without finding a way to enable Sari to engage in the process.

Alert

Being alert implies aware, accountable engagement with service users which avoids the dangers of routinised, procedure-led practice. Practice should not be something which we sleepwalk through – it should be an active encounter with people who may be disadvantaged on a number of levels. We should be alert to potential areas for discrimination and oppression, including our own personal beliefs and values and those of the organisations in which we work. The risk for practitioners is that we can become so overwhelmed by the pressures of the daily workload and the organisational targets and pressures that, unless we make a conscious choice to be vigilant, self-aware and critical, in the sense of being consciously aware of the need to question the taken-for-granted, that we may forget that our primary aim is to help people, and that the purpose of what we do is to meet the needs and respect the rights of individuals who use services (Adams *et al.* 2009).

In relation to the case study, alert practice is being demonstrated by the reflections and involvement of the practitioners concerned. Rather than just accepting the situation they are actively engaged in trying to look behind the way the problem is being presented (old lady with physical medical problem) and using their professional knowledge and experience to analyse critically what this situation could mean for this particular person.

Reflective

Reflective practice is taught throughout health and social work/care education. This is the domain where the practitioner becomes aware of how her or his own feelings, beliefs and values can affect the way in which they engage with service users and carry out their practice. Schon (1983) talks about the processes of *reflection-in-action* where the professional responds to a situation almost without being aware of the knowledge, skills and values he or she is employing. Schon calls this 'instinctive' practice or 'tacit knowledge' which accumulates within practitioners through experience and which can be called on in a wide variety of situations. While this can be very useful, Schon also talks about the importance of *reflection-on-action* where the professional, away from the pressures of everyday work, gets the opportunity to think through their practice in a way that is more critical and objective. Greaves and Yardley in Chapter 4 highlight the importance of supervision for practitioners working with child protection but it is clear that anyone working in emotional and uncertain situations with people who are vulnerable or at risk would benefit from space to think about their practice.

In complex situations like the one discussed in the case study, room for critical reflection is particularly important in order to provide the opportunity to weigh up the various elements that might be going on in relation to rights, risks and responsibilities. Not to do so could lead to the kind of outcome that happened before, where the wishes and views of the person at the centre of the process may have been marginalised or ignored (even with good intent) because she does not have the power to insist that her voice be heard.

Empowering

Empowerment is one of those words used so frequently and with such a variety of meanings that it has almost become a cliché within health and social care. And yet an understanding of how power can be used or misused within the situations we encounter is absolutely vital if the needs and rights of service users are to be addressed effectively. Much of the time practitioners feel that they have very little power and that it is their managers, their colleagues or even service users themselves who have the power but this is to misunderstand the nature of what empowerment can achieve and how oppressive the lack of empowering practice can feel to those using health and social work services.

Neil Thompson's book *Power and Empowerment* (2007) provides a useful introduction to theories of power and empowerment, and how these can be applied in real situations to promote change through empowering practice. He highlights the importance of working in partnership with people who use services and proposes a new kind of professionalism, where power is genuinely shared between professionals and service users. There have been ongoing attempts to shift some power towards people who use services in health and social care, and this aspect of practice remains highly relevant in respect of forthcoming changes in provision of health and social care and the Personalisation agenda. The case study above, however, demonstrates how easily the social worker and the carers assumed they knew what was best for Sari Vishnamurthi and because of the power dynamics in that situation she did not feel able to challenge the decisions that were made.

Dynamic

Particularly in areas of risk and where the practitioner is unsure of how to work though a situation of complexity and uncertainty, the principle of maintaining a dynamic approach is vital. Often practitioners have so much else demanded of them that the more difficult situation can be allowed to drift, leaving vulnerable adults or children at risk of being ignored or let down by the system. Being dynamic does not always mean 'doing something' – in fact PREPARED practice may also be about not intervening in a situation where people have the right or responsibility to manage a risky situation in their own way. But it is not just about 'leaving them to it'. If there is to be a risk assessment, it needs to be a dynamic process involving the service user and relevant stakeholders, and if the decision is made that intervention is not advisable or possible, it needs to be a positive decision, not one that is reached by default.

Applying the PREPARED model

No model can encompass all the complexities of practice but having such a model can help us to be consciously aware of the constituents of good practice. This model offers an opportunity for practitioners to think constructively about their relationships with each other and with service users and all the other stakeholders who may be involved in the case of a particular individual who uses health or social care services. The world outside practice, which does not recognise the complexity involved, continues to expect that somehow it should be possible to balance perfectly the relationships between rights and risks, autonomy and capacity, vulnerability and choice. While these expectations will continue to challenge the best intentions of critical and conscientious practitioners, all professionals will need to be acutely aware of their own values and attitudes, the knowledge, powers and responsibilities they hold and share, and the significance of these for promoting or inhibiting the rights and responsibilities of the vulnerable people (and their carers and networks) who they encounter in their professional capacity.

Conclusion

Looking closely at the findings of Serious Case Reviews and listening to the testimonies of practitioners from a range of professional backgrounds has highlighted that some of the most difficult and perplexing dilemmas rest on finding a way to achieve the impossible – to perfectly balance the tensions between rights, risks and responsibilities. This book has drawn on the experience of individuals from a range of professional backgrounds to seek out theories, models and perspectives to help manage this complex and ever-changing balance. This is appropriate as one of the key findings of all the investigations is the importance of good interprofessional working. For practitioners this means a clear understanding of our own and others' roles and responsibilities, duties and accountabilities, professional requirements and the expectations of the public.

However, even in writing the book it became clear that the external pressures from the media, for example, can lead to risk-averse perspectives which err on the side of caution and which could rather limit the opportunities for people who use services, rather than risk-aware practice which recognises the problems that may arise but would rather work alongside people, emphasising rights and strengths whenever possible. Clearly there are some people – some children, some very frail adults – in such risky situations that clear action and decisive intervention must be carried out in a timely manner. However, it is also important to remember that for many people who use health and social care services, the process can easily lead to increased disability and dependency, often by people who may feel they have the person's 'best interests' at heart. It is not by accident that we chose to start this book by looking at peoples' rights, and it is not by chance that the PREPARED model focuses so heavily on the rights, choices and wishes of people who use services. It is because in the uncertain future faced by health and welfare services, and by those who work in them and those who depend on them, we need models which offer frameworks for working equitably in partnership with colleagues and service users in an attempt to achieve the most appropriate balance in the shifting landscape of rights, risks and responsibilities.

Further reading

Hothersall, S. J. and Maas-Lowitt, M. (eds) (2010) *Need, Risk and Protection in Social Work Practice*. Exeter: Learning Matters.

Johns, R. (2009) *Using the Law in Social Work* (4th edn). Exeter: Learning Matters.

Johns, R. (2011) *Social Work, Social Policy and Older People*. Exeter: Learning Matters.

SCIE (2010) *Personalisation Briefing – Better Knowledge for Better Practice Implications for Social Workers in Adult Services*. SCIE Report 29, October, online.

Shakespeare, T. (2000) *Help*. London: British Association of Social Workers.

Smith, D. (ed.) (2004) *Social Work and Evidence-Based Practice*. London: Jessica Kingsley.

References

Adams, R., Dominelli, L. and Payne, M. (eds) (2009) *Critical Practice in Social Work* (2nd edn). Basingstoke: Palgrave Macmillan.

Armstrong, J. (2008) *The Scottish Legislation: The Way Forward?* In T. Mantell and A. Scragg (eds), *Safeguarding Adults in Social Work*. Exeter: Learning Matters.

Association of Directors of Adult Services (2005) *Safeguarding Adults: A National Framework of Standards for Good Practice in Adult Protection Work*. London: ADSS.

Banks, S. (2006) *Ethics and Values in Social Work* (3rd edn). Basingstoke: Palgrave Macmillan.

Bowles, W., Collingwood, M., Curry, S. and Valentine, B. (2006) *Ethical Practice in Social Work*. Maidenhead: McGraw Hill/Open University Press.

Brammer, A. (2010) *Social Work Law* (3rd edn). Harlow: Pearson Education.

Brown, K. (ed.) (2010) *Vulnerable Adults and Community Care* (2nd edn). Exeter: Learning Matters.

Currer, C. (2007) *Loss and Social Work*. Exeter: Learning Matters.

Department of Health (1998) *Who Decides?* London: HMSO.

Department of Health (2000) *No Secrets*. London: Department of Health.

Department of Health (2009) *Safeguarding Adults: A Consultation on the Review on 'No Secrets' Guidance*. London: Department of Health.

Dominelli, L. (2002) *Anti-oppressive Social Work Theory and Practice*. Basingstoke: Palgrave Macmillan.

Flynn, M. (2007) *The Murder of Steven Hoskin: A Serious Case Review – Executive Summary*. Cornwall: Adult Protection Committee.

Fook, J. and Gardner, F. (2010) *Practising Critical Reflection*. Maidenhead: McGraw Hill/Open University Press.

Galpin, D. and Bates, N. (2009) *Social Work Practice with Adults*. Exeter: Learning Matters.

Gray, M. and Webb, S. A. (eds) (2010) *Ethics and Value Perspectives in Social Work*. Basingstoke: Palgrave Macmillan.

Hek, G. and Moule, P. (2006) *Making Sense of Research: An Introduction for Health and Social Care Practitioners* (3rd edn). London: Sage.

Jasper, M. (2006) *Reflection, Professional Judgement and Decision-making*. Oxford: Blackwell.

Johns, R. (2007) Who decides now? Protecting and empowering vulnerable adults who lose capacity to make decisions for themselves. *British Journal of Social Work*, 37(3): 557–64.

Kitwood, T. (1997) *Dementia Reconsidered: The Person Comes First*. Buckingham: Open University Press.

Koubel, G. and Bungay, H. (eds) (2009) *The Challenge of Person-Centred Care: Interprofessional Perspectives*. Basingstoke: Palgrave Macmillan.

Laird, S. (2008) *Anti Oppressive Social Work: A Guide for Developing Cultural Competence*. London: Sage.

Martin, J. (2007) *Safeguarding Adults*. Lyme Regis: Russell House.

Morris, J. (1997) *Community Care: Working in Partnership with Service Users*. Birmingham: Venture Press.

Newman, T., Moseley, A., Tierney, S. and Ellis, A. (2005) *Evidence-based Social Work*. Lyme Regis: Russell House.

Schon, D. (1983) *The Reflective Practitioner: How Professionals Think in Action*. New York: Basic Books.

Scragg, A. and Mantell, T. (eds) (2011) *Safeguarding Adults in Social Work* (2nd edn). Exeter: Learning Matters.

Swain, J., French, S. and Cameron, C. (2005) *Controversial Issues in a Disabling Society*. Maidenhead: McGraw Hill//Open University.

Thompson, N. (2007) *Power and Empowerment*. Lyme Regis: Russell House.

CHAPTER 12

Conclusion

Georgina Koubel

The main objective of this book is to help those within health and social care to think more carefully, critically and creatively about practice with people who may be seen as vulnerable because they use services. Previous chapters have helped to consider how complex and contested are the factors that impact on the balance of rights, risks and responsibilities of those working with vulnerable people in health and social care, as well as those of service users themselves. This conclusion will highlight the themes that have emerged and explore their significance for practitioners.

One factor that emerges from many of the accounts is the over-concern about risk, perhaps at the expense of consideration of the other two elements, the rights of service users and the various responsibilities of the practitioners and those individuals and families who use health and welfare services. One of the reasons for this must be the impact of the media in highlighting where mistakes have been made. While there are many lessons to be learned from each of these undoubted tragedies, and it is crucial that we address them as thoroughly as possible without being defensive, the scapegoating of professionals – most notably but by no means exclusively social workers – does have a tendency to lead to the risk of over-cautious or risk-averse practice (Titterton 2005).

There appears to be a view, particularly in relation to people with mental health difficulties or those who misuse substances, that issues of risk coincide with issues of dangerousness (Ryan and Pritchard 2004). One of the features of a social model of risk, that is, one that locates risk in context and complexity rather than within the individual or as a result of their impairments, is that it tries to dispel myths and stereotypes and replace these with a model that respects and supports individuals as far as possible, intervening only when it is manifestly in the best interests of the individual. However, it has also become evident from the findings of serious case reviews that in some situations involving either children or vulnerable adults that health and social care services have not intervened as quickly as we should have, and that at times we have left vulnerable individuals to deal alone with extremely challenging and sometimes fatal circumstances.

The discourses that have been explored in this book have grappled with the dilemmas that face practitioners who need to discharge their professional responsibilities while adhering to principles of anti-oppressive practice. It is difficult and probably unproductive to try to find any one single model of risk that can manage all challenges. Different models of risk may be applicable within different contexts and with different groups of service users. The encounter between professionals and practitioners from health and social care and service users not infrequently encompasses elements of control as well as a requirement to advocate and support the rights and choices of individuals. Social care and health professionals work together at the borderline between the challenge of empowerment and the duty to protect. Personal and professional values impact significantly on our attitudes towards how we manage this tension (Pritchard 2001; Braye and Preston-Shoot 1995).

Another requirement of the professional role is how we move towards finding a balance between the rights and needs of different parties to the process of intervention. This book has looked at different ways of thinking about rights, risks and the personal and professional (including essentially interprofessional) responsibilities that inform practice in health and social care. Throughout the text we have offered challenges and case studies that enable reflection around the complexities of working with both children and families and adults and their networks in the context of policy and practice developments. One way to address these issues is to look at how the relationship between the state and the individual is changing, and try to understand how this will affect the relationship of the balance in relation to rights, risks and responsibilities for practitioners in health and social care.

Looking back – looking ahead

Looking back, we have apparently come a long way in a comparatively short space of time. In working with people with learning or physical disabilities, a few decades have seen considerable changes in the lived experience of those people who use services. One key factor is the recognition that terms like 'vulnerability' and 'disability' reflect not an objective reality but a construction of how people are perceived and valued within society (Fook 2002).

In 1998 it was identified that there was a need for an official framework for deciding who should have the right – and the responsibility – of making decisions for those adults who were unable to make them for themselves (Department of Health 1998). The assumption at that time was that whoever was in closest proximity to the person had the right to decide what was best for them. Now there is a whole system dedicated to ensuring that adults who may be considered vulnerable but who are capable of understanding and making their own decisions do not have this right taken away.

Differences between adults and children's services

Issues of need, risk and protection continue to challenge practitioners in health and social care (Hothersall and Maas-Lowit 2010) and we have to continue to look for models and guides that can help intervene in risky and uncertain situations. In working with children at risk, there are many challenges but there is at least a clear legal framework for intervention in cases where children may need to be removed from situations where they are deemed to be 'at risk of significant harm' (Children Act 1989, 2004) whether or not the children or their families are happy or willing to accept that intervention.

While there are some statutory instruments relating to adults such as the *No Secrets* (Department of Health 2000) requirement that all local authorities should implement multi-agency adult protection policies and procedures and the Protection of Vulnerable Groups Act 2006, which addresses the vetting and barring of people who work with adults at risk, there is at present no specific law as there is for children that can enable workers to intervene with an adult with capacity who refuses to cooperate. Learning from cases such as those of Victoria Climbié has led to the development of increasingly sophisticated models of assessment, including risk assessment. Social workers in Children and Families' Services understandably feel additional pressure from the media about their concern for the children they seek to support and protect, and it is possible that this pressure will not decrease as resources become less widely available.

For adults who use services, the future is very hard to read. Some strategies, such as reducing or removing disability benefits and limiting the availability of local authority or voluntary organisations' resources, might appear to augur less choice and independence for some people with learning and physical disabilities, while, on the other hand, the introduction of Personalisation which has given many a greater degree of independence following its introduction by the previous government (Carr and Dittrich 2008; SCIE 2010) seems to mesh quite nicely with the Coalition Government's avowed aim to reduce dependency on the state and to place greater responsibility and control back in the hands of the individual.

However, a number of tragedies have also befallen adults at risk, although these do not always attract the attention of the media or the public as do those of children. In some cases it is a matter of people who have no power and who are perhaps not regarded highly by the public at large who are let down, damaged and even killed by the very services that are meant to be helping them. Whether these people have mental capacity or not is irrelevant. They are made vulnerable not because they are old, sick or disabled but by the attitudes and values of others and the lack of power or influence to affect their own situations. One finding of all these reports is crystal clear. Whether the people found to have been harmed have mental capacity or not, it is the attitudes and values of those around them which need to change. Whether current government policies will enhance or inhibit the integration of vulnerable adults into society remains to be seen.

The challenge for practitioners is to remain on high alert to the changes and their implications for vulnerable service users. One way to do this is to think about the models presented in this book, and the various perspectives that have been examined and to share your experiences with other practitioners to find ways to assess and protect where necessary without compromising the rights of the people who use services to be protected from abuse while still living fulfilling lives. This means that however the systems develop to measure and contain risk, the person who is being assessed has to remain at the heart of the process (Koubel and Bungay 2009).

The PREPARED model is not a risk assessment model as such but may be useful as a guide for maintaining value-based, ethical practice in the face of whatever changes the ideological winds blow in. Sometimes good intentions are not enough, and we need the rigour of placing the rights of individuals at the heart of our considerations and interventions, as well as being mindful of the roles, risks and responsibilities involved in interprofessional practice.

Further reading

Thompson, N. (2007) *Power and Empowerment*. Lyme Regis: Russell House.
Thompson, S. (2005) *Age Discrimination*. Lyme Regis: Russell House.

References

Braye, S. and Preston-Shoot, M. (1995) *Empowering Practice in Health and Social Care*. Open University Press.
Carr, S. and Dittrich, R. (2008) *Personalisation: A Rough Guide*. London: Social Care Institute of Excellence.
Department of Health (1998) *Who Decides?* London: HMSO.
Department of Health (2000) *No Secrets*. London: Department of Health.
Fook, J. (2002) *Social Work: Critical Theory and Practice*. London: Sage.
Hothersall, S. J. and Maas-Lowit, M. (eds) (2010) *Need, Risk and Protection in Social Work Practice*. Exeter: Learning Matters.
Koubel, G. and Bungay, H. (eds) (2009) *The Challenge of Person-Centred Care: An Interprofessional Perspective*. Basingstoke: Palgrave Macmillan.
Pritchard, J. (2001) *Good Practice with Vulnerable Adults*. London: Jessica Kingsley.
Ryan, T. and Pritchard, J. (2004) (eds) *Good Practice in Adult Mental Health*. London: Jessica Kingsley.
SCIE (2010) *Personalisation Briefing – Better Knowledge for Better Practice Implications for Social Workers in Adults Services*. Report 29, October. London: Social Care Institute of Excellence.
Titterton, M. (2005) *Risk and Risk Taking in Health and Social Welfare*. London: Jessica Kingsley.

Index

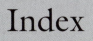